TAKE CHARGE
of Your HEALTHCARE
MANAGEMENT CAREER

TAKE
CHARGE
of Your HEALTHCARE
MANAGEMENT CAREER

50
Lessons That
Drive Success

Kenneth R. White and J. Stephen Lindsey

AUPHA

Health Administration Press, Chicago, Illinois
Association of University Programs in Health Administration, Arlington, Virginia

Library of Congress Cataloging-in-Publication Data

White, Kenneth R. (Kenneth Ray), 1956– , author.
  Take charge of your healthcare management career : 50 lessons that drive success / Kenneth R. White and J. Stephen Lindsey.
    p. ; cm.
  Includes bibliographical references.
  ISBN 978-1-56793-692-6 (alk. paper)
  I. Lindsey, J. Stephen, author. II. Association of University Programs in Health Administration, publisher. III. Title.
  [DNLM: 1. Health Facility Administrators. 2. Career Mobility. 3. Health Services Administration. WX 155]
  RA971.35
  362.10683—dc23
                              2014035846

The paper used in this publication meets the minimum requirements of American National Standard for Information Sciences—Permanence of Paper for Printed Library Materials, ANSI Z39.48-1984.∞™

Acquisitions editor: Janet Davis; Project editor: Andrew Baumann; Cover designer: Brad Norr; Layout: PerfecType.

Found an error or a typo? We want to know! Please e-mail it to hapbooks@ache.org, and put "Book Error" in the subject line.

For photocopying and copyright information, please contact Copyright Clearance Center at www.copyright.com or at (978) 750-8400.

Health Administration Press
A division of the Foundation of the American
   College of Healthcare Executives
One North Franklin Street, Suite 1700
Chicago, IL 60606-3529
(312) 424-2800

Association of University Programs
   in Health Administration
2000 North 14th Street
Suite 780
Arlington, VA 22201
(703) 894-0940

To our students past, present, and future, and all the lessons you've taught us. To the joy of being part of a profession that gives us all the opportunity to do what is best for the patient.

Contents

Acknowledgments

FIRST AND FOREMOST, we acknowledge each other for the joy of working together for many years in the service of teaching and developing others in our healthcare administration profession. This book is a vision that developed over several years during our conversations about how we can help new generations of healthcare executives succeed in our profession. We have learned from each other, supported each other, and, in the process, deepened a friendship.

Several of our colleagues read early drafts of certain lessons and contributed wisdom and suggestions for the book. These individuals are Dr. Jim Begun, Pat Cleary, Hud Connery, Brian Cook, Terrie Edwards, Pat Farrell, Alan Hiss, Sam Jordan, Joyce Kennedy, Dell Oliver, Will Wagnon, and Dana Williams. Several people contributed to specific lessons: Maury Denton (Lesson 2), Barrett Clark (Lesson 28), Brent Higgins (Lesson 38), John Mitchell (Lesson 46), and Ed Landry (Lesson 50).

Each of the 50 lessons starts with a quote from a practitioner or expert on the subject of the lesson. We owe a debt of gratitude to the people who gave of their time and expertise to review the lessons and provide quotes. Many improvements resulted from their input.

We are grateful for the opportunity to work together in leading the Master of Health Administration program at Virginia Commonwealth University (VCU) and for the privilege of working with students and alumni who have a passion for healthcare management and leadership. We thank the VCU colleagues from whom we received support and encouragement—especially Dr. Steve Mick, Dr. Dolores Clement, Dr. Bob Hurley, Dr. Shirley Gibson, Dr. Mark Diana, Suzanne Havasy, and many others.

We are deeply appreciative of two expert editors—Christine Kueter and Suzie Bird. Christine edited the entire book and blended the lessons into a single voice. Without this expertise, we daresay the book would have been much more difficult to send to press. We are also grateful to Janet Davis, Drew Baumann, and their colleagues at Health Administration Press, who believed in our concept for this book, encouraged us to stretch, and supported us every step of the way.

I (Ken) thank my spouse, Dr. Carl Outen, for his support, encouragement, and patience while I was writing the book. Also, thanks to Dean Dorrie Fontaine of the University of Virginia School of Nursing, who supports our work in many ways and under whose vision and leadership I am allowed to grow professionally. Sister Julie Hyer, OP, has been a steadfast friend and mentor since 1980, has provided counsel and ideas, and has served as a sounding board. For more than 20 years, Dr. Norma Geddes has inspired me "to follow my bliss."

I (Steve) thank my loving wife Miriam, who read and proofed much of the material for the book, and I acknowledge the inspiration I received about leadership and management from business guru and writer Peter Drucker. Also, special thanks to the partners at Ivy Ventures for their understanding, encouragement, and support of this project. Robyn O'Neil of Ivy Ventures has provided support in countless ways over the years. Dr. Edward Martirosian, president of the board of directors of HCA Henrico Doctors' Hospital, has been a friend and mentor since 1979. Many leadership ideas were formed by my early experience in the US Army and at HCA. Dr. Thomas Frist Sr., Dr. Thomas Frist Jr., and Jack Bovender of HCA have all served as role models.

Introduction

IT GOES WITHOUT saying that no perfect job exists. No organization, group of people, or position on earth comes without some measure of challenges, problems, and messiness. But there are ways to deal with the world's near-constant imperfections, particularly in the workplace, and certain universal truths make it possible to find best practices and answers. So with those observations in mind, and with more than eight decades of professional experience between us, we've compiled 50 lessons to steer you thoughtfully, carefully, and with poise and grace toward, onto, and along your chosen career path as a healthcare manager.

This book aims to introduce the early careerist to healthcare management by taking a three-pronged approach. The organization of the book into a trio of themes—Manage Yourself, Manage Your Job, and Take Charge of Your Career—is based on the refrains we heard from puzzled health administration students, frustrated hiring managers, and exasperated company executives who butted heads, roiled in misunderstandings, and allowed egos and narcissism to trump best practices. Most of us can benefit from recalibrations such as returning to basic self-awareness, fervently desiring to make things better and to learn to pay attention to what matters most, and matching our gifts, talents, and experience with the right organization and role.

Life, work, and everything in between should be informed by these ideas. Those who dismiss them likely won't perform well or contribute to their organization's mission, vision, and values. They may be overlooked for promotions and find it difficult to move elsewhere, even laterally. They may be outsourced, outmoded, and outmaneuvered by others.

Success isn't something you're born with; it's carefully cultivated, mastered, and honed. The most successful healthcare executives have learned that authenticity and truth are the best path, and they have learned to *really* pay attention, to *truly* be consummate professionals, and to *wholly* be the very best version of themselves that they can be. The traits, lessons, and skills outlined in this book must be mastered for maximum personal, career, and work success.

We all have dream jobs—those positions that lie at the intersection of our gifts, our passions, and the needs of society. When it works well, a job can fit like a glove and be satisfying to one's very core. We hope that this book and its lessons will help you find the kind of professional joy you're seeking.

We wish you the best.

Ken White and Steve Lindsey
Richmond, Virginia

Manage Yourself

WHY START A book on careers with a section on how to manage yourself? It's always best, as Glinda the Good Witch says in *The Wizard of Oz*, to start at the beginning. If you can't manage yourself, you can't tackle all the things that come next: people and budgets, the complaint of a patient's family, or your own business. If you don't have a realistic picture of your strengths, gifts, and talents or don't know what you need to learn and how to present yourself as a professional, you can't make your very best leap out of the starting gate.

Of course, plenty of people don't follow the lessons that are detailed in this section. They're the ones who have never cultivated an interest in others and remain determined narcissists; the managers who are so risk averse that they're ineffective; the individuals who overly rely on technology for their presentations, then hit snags and become utterly derailed; the people who misuse social media to their detriment or who cast blame rather than own their mistakes; and those whose speech, writing, and presentation skills lull audiences into a stupor.

Those who aren't familiar with Lessons 1–18 sometimes commit gaffes that are almost too bad to be true. For example, the graduate student who sent her job application in a mailing tube with her résumé on pink scented paper, a glamour shot picture, and a return e-mail address that contained the word *diva*; the former colleague who, although smart and well educated, talked too familiarly and revealed too much; the peer who whined, complained, and always lamented why something *couldn't* be done and who wondered why people avoided her; or the practitioner who was so burned out that he brought others—including his patients—down with him.

These individuals never bothered to look at themselves to figure out why others reacted to them so strongly, why they remained ineffective in their jobs, why colleagues avoided them, and why, ultimately, their positions were eliminated or they were fired. They didn't take the time to manage *themselves* first.

When you manage *yourself* and cultivate the best *you* there is, good things happen. Then you're like the hospital CEO who visited us in a hospital other than his own when we were ill; like the colleagues who jotted notes of thanks to us for small things, tucking them in our mailboxes or under our doors; like the coworkers who sent food, flowers, or plants when a relative died; and like those who listened intently, compassionately, and with the kind of interest that today is all too rare.

So much of who we are at a job begins with who and how we are as humans. It's important to know what to do and what not to do—and although some lessons in this section may seem obvious, they're important enough to spell out explicitly. The lessons for success in this section will get you off to a good start in taking charge of your career.

Establish a Life Vision

A career decision based on the expectations of others
will be unrewarding. Listen to your heart. Choose a role
that yields personal fulfillment. If you are engaged in
something with purpose, the payoff will be generous.

—*Beth Merchent, MHA, MBA,*
vice president of community health services,
Bon Secours Virginia Health System, Richmond

SO YOU'VE GOT the academic training, your degree(s), and perhaps an internship or two behind you—and you have the hun-
ger for a life-changing career in healthcare management. Now's
the perfect time to establish a personal vision statement for your
career—just as though you were developing a campaign or a slogan
to market a company's assets, only this time, it's all about *you*.

It's crucial to begin your professional journey by taking an honest look at yourself—what you're like, what your strengths are, what
others say about you—and then mapping out a series of goals to
declare a vision for your professional life. Jotting down notes is a
good way to begin. This document doesn't have to be formal or
intensive, but spend some time and thought on it. Following are a
few questions to consider to get you started:

- What do you value most?
- How do you like to spend your day?

- What have others told you you're good at? What do *you* consider your strengths to be?
- How do you want to make a difference in the world?
- Where do you want to be in 5, 10, or 20 years?
- What's your ideal job, and where?
- What sort of leader would you like to be?
- How would you like to be remembered?

Remember not to rely exclusively on outside sources for advice that will determine your future—look inside yourself. Ask yourself what makes you happy. Record your thoughts over time, and you may find a path for your career. *You* may have the best career advice in your soul.

Remember, too, that your personal vision statement is a fluid document. You're not a slave to it; rather, you can change it as you see fit. As you progress in your career, different ideas will occur to you—new or additional educational goals, hopes for geographic change, determination to broaden your experience in one direction versus another—and it's wise to keep your personal vision statement up to date as your thoughts about your trajectory shift.

Like a physical exam or dental checkup, schedule regular meetings with yourself to consider (or reconsider) your vision statement. From time to time, make sure it still works for you.

EXERCISE 1

Think of some defining moments in your life—times, choices, or situations that have defined who you are today. For each defining moment, articulate how it shaped your values. How do these instances inform your life vision? What will you be doing, and what impact do you want to make on the world in, say, 30 years?

EXERCISE 2

It's the day of your funeral. Three people will each deliver a short eulogy on your life and the impact you made. One will offer thoughts on your work life, one will share thoughts of your family and friends, and one will speak about your contribution to the world. What do you hope they will say?

RESOURCES

Palmer, P. J. 2009. *A Hidden Wholeness: The Journey Toward an Undivided Life.* San Francisco: Jossey-Bass.

————. 2000. *Let Your Life Speak: Listening for the Voice of Vocation.* San Francisco: Jossey-Bass.

Get Comfortable with Risk

Innovation is about pushing the envelope, where execution is the
vanguard to overcome the inevitable challenges and obstacles
along the way. If there is no chance of failure, the endeavor
is not true innovation. Taking calculated risks and having a
willingness to learn from mistakes is necessary.

—*Brent Higgins, MHA,*
bundled payment director, WellPoint Inc.,
Richmond, Virginia

DURING MILITARY TRAINING, a sergeant will scream, "Make a
decision, lieutenant!" What the sergeant means is: Gather as many
facts as possible in the time you have and then give it your best
shot—because lives may be at stake. This is a call to action.

The call translates to civilian life, too. Be prepared to take a few
big risks in your career, particularly early on. Think about starting
a company or joining a start-up. Many successful executives began
their professional lives by taking a job that stretched their capabili-
ties and found that the process ultimately advanced their careers.

Note that, in this fast-paced world, doing nothing is inherently
risky. We often consider the risk and consequences of our actions,
but we should also remember that the status quo and inaction also
carry huge risks.

Risks are a necessary part of any job—and to be a successful
healthcare executive, you'll need to get really comfortable with

them. It's simply a fact that those who learn to take calculated risks that align with their organization's goals and vision will achieve better results throughout their career. Although the safe road feels more comfortable, change is the only constant in healthcare organizations—and those organizations are, without exception, looking for leaders who can get results. That means mastering the route to change.

Taking risks, however, does not mean acting recklessly. Think about what will happen *after* you take the leap, whatever it might be. Talk to people you trust, and get their take. Make sure you have both capital and time enough to pivot onto the next project, should things go awry. Weigh the chances of success, and make sure you have what you need to make your leap a success. With all that in place, you are ready to take a risk.

Successful entrepreneurs sometimes advise, "Fail small and fail fast." When you first observe a problem, think of it as an opportunity. Ask yourself how you can solve it and what product or procedure might be part of the solution.

Also remember the value in speaking up. When your team is struggling with a problem, do you offer the solution that you have been considering? Or do you hold back and wait for someone else to suggest it? Many former executives say that their only regrets center around not being more forceful and vocal in offering their opinions and ideas when faced with seemingly insurmountable problems. Speaking up is essential, even if your idea doesn't feel fully baked.

Remember, too, the element of time. Many executives tend to overestimate risk when they maneuver into new or unknown areas. Fear of failure and fear of the unknown can lead to inaction precisely when action is what's required.

As you weigh your options, remember: No decision has a 100 percent guaranteed chance of success—but standing still in healthcare is never an option either.

Here are steps to follow when taking risks:

1. **Understand exactly what problem you're trying to solve.** Spend time defining the central problem or issue.

2. **Gather information and facts about the problem.** Once the problem has been determined, gather information. Talk to people and listen carefully. Analyze and discuss potential solutions in a thoughtful, organized way.

3. **Identify the best course of action.** Once potential solutions have been considered, decide who should have a hand in solving it. What do they see as the best possible solution? Listen carefully and thoughtfully, and be amenable to tweaking the solution based on what others advise.

4. **Consider the possible outcomes or consequences of your risk.** What's the best result your decision might bring? What's the worst? Learn to project scenarios that may unfold from your decision, remembering to consider legal, budgetary, and regulatory issues.

5. **Go for it.** When you have about 80 percent of your questions answered, take the risk. In the risk's early days, take time to analyze your results.

6. **Encourage others on your staff to take risks, too.** Doing so will instill a level of strategic thinking in your organization's culture.

Those who offer solutions and are not afraid to speak out develop a reputation as problem solvers—the kind of people whom healthcare organizations value highly. Although you will make mistakes, remember to learn from them to improve your rate of success. Remind yourself that you are in the healthcare field to make a difference, solve problems, and improve things. Be that executive who gets things done—not the one who gets outmoded because you kept silent at a critical juncture.

EXERCISE 1

Whether it's a household, personal, or work problem, set a goal to understand and devise a solution to an issue that you currently face within the next 30 days.

EXERCISE 2

Keep a personal journal of your decisions. Assign a risk to each decision you make. Then, later, go back and look at your decisions. What could you have done to improve your chances for success? Periodically review your journal. Are you improving in your ability to assess problems and take risks?

RESOURCE

Clark, B., and S. Lindsey. 2013. "Success Requires Risk: 5 Ways Health System Leaders Should Undertake Risk and Uncertainty to Succeed." *Becker's Hospital Review.* Published November 25. www.beckershospitalreview.com /hospital-management-administration/success-requires -risk-5-ways-health-system-leaders-should-undertake-risk -and-uncertainty-to-succeed.html.

Focus Your Time

The best leaders motivate and engage the organization by demonstrating a personal ability to deliver on promises in a timely fashion—but show confidence and trust in employees' abilities as well. As leaders, we must delegate and hold others accountable. We must trust and verify. Investing time in others, clearly communicating expectations, and keeping away from time-wasting activities are critical ingredients of every healthcare CEO. Proper time management also means knowing what can be deleted or ignored—and what truly rises to the top.

—Jackie DeSouza, MHA,
CEO, Research Medical Center,
HCA Midwest Health System,
Kansas City, Missouri

A MAJOR THIEF of your success is inappropriate management of your time. What does wasted time look like? Like a lot of things you see every day in offices across America: Pointless hallway conversations. Aimless Internet surfing. Procrastination. Texting with friends and family. Failing to manage your electronic files and having a disorganized, jumbled computer desktop. Overly long lunches without a work focus.

However, you can lose time in other, not so obvious ways. Time can be wasted by taking on too much or by planning wholly unrealistic project deadlines. Because time is money, as they say, as well as something you need to build your career, perhaps the most subtle time waster is working on things that will not give you the best return.

Daniel Goleman, author of *Focus: The Hidden Driver of Excellence,* asserts that our digital era has caused us to be more engaged with machines than with the people around us—a circumstance that has also blunted our ability to pay attention and maintain focus. Attention is a critical ingredient in managing your time; you need it to prioritize the projects that lie before you, to zero in on the tasks at hand, and to fully deliver on promises and expectations. Without it, you're just another time waster, and the world is rife with those.

So, what can you do to best manage your time?

- **Practice being focused and attentive.** Tackling a task that requires lengthy, sustained attention—or listening thoughtfully to a colleague, your spouse, or your partner—is a great way to sharpen this skill, which is a critical first step to fighting off time wasters.

- **Limit your goals.** Focus your (and your team's) energy on a few important projects and goals that you can execute well. Don't volunteer to take on new projects or goals that are so many or so diverse that you can't do any of them well. Choose a few, if you're able, and dig in so you can knock them out of the park.

- **Be organized from the get-go.** Although metal filing cabinets have today been replaced by computers, many people's electronic files are as messy, poorly organized, and difficult to navigate as those hulking rows of steel. Is your desktop littered with old, useless photos and files that need to be trashed? Do you have hundreds of thousands of old e-mails from years back? Take the time to clean up. Develop a system to file, back up, and share information. Nothing is more maddening—or a bigger waste of your time—than not being able to locate what you need when you need it. Develop a system to organize yourself at the project's start.

- **Teach, empower, and delegate.** The old adage "If you want something done right, do it yourself" is a time waster. Teaching others how to handle a task may require more time up front, but empowering them by delegating is key to effective time management. Showing confidence in others by delegating important projects to them is also a natural means of cultivating loyalty and trust among your colleagues and employees. If you're surrounded by capable people, they'll be glad for your vote of confidence and will likely be eager to please you.

- **Group similar activities together during your day, and set a limited amount of time to work on them.** Schedule regular slots of time to check e-mail, return phone calls, work on particular projects, and make rounds. Always carry a notepad or electronic device when away from your desk so that you can jot down notes and reminders to yourself. However, don't become a slave to your device in the name of being organized—know when to put it down so that you can, as a healthcare manager, be attuned and attentive to your many stakeholders.

- **Understand that complications and disruptions happen.** In healthcare, no day goes exactly according to plan. However, you can accommodate the inevitable ups and downs by planning in advance. Assign yourself "soft" deadlines. If a report is due on May 15, your deadline should be May 1. That will give you adequate time to deal with any disruptions that may crop up.

- **Focus on activities that add value to your organization's mission.** Generally, for healthcare organizations, value is related to improving patients' health and sustaining the health of caregivers. As you lead meetings, read e-mails, and write reports, ask yourself how these activities contribute—in ways big and small, direct and indirect—to the overall mission of your organization. That alone will give you a sense of what is truly important in your work and what deserves most of your attention.

EXERCISE 1

Divide your tasks into a half dozen or so subject areas (with headings that reflect your role and responsibilities in your organization, e.g., *meetings, correspondence, finances, special projects, human resources*), then keep track of how you spend your day in each area. As you log your day, acknowledge what might be improved by identifying the thieves of your time. At the end of the day, how can you be a better steward of your time—and thus of your career?

EXERCISE 2

Using Stephen Covey's book, *The 7 Habits of Highly Effective People,* identify what is urgent or important, and reprioritize your daily activities.

RESOURCES

Birkinshaw, J., and J. Cohen. 2013. "Make Time for the Work That Matters." *Harvard Business Review* 91 (9): 115–18.

Covey, S. R. 2013. *The 7 Habits of Highly Effective People: Powerful Lessons in Personal Change,* anniversary edition. New York: Simon & Schuster.

Duhigg, C. 2012. *The Power of Habit: Why We Do What We Do in Life and Business.* New York: Random House.

Goleman, D. 2013. *Focus: The Hidden Driver of Excellence.* New York: HarperCollins.

Adopt Appreciative Practice

Positive connections among members of a team, unit, or organization promote resilience and creativity in response to emerging and unpredictable future challenges. Appreciative practice is a formal tool for creating positive connections. Seek out others in your team, unit, or organization who have done good work and compliment them. Better yet, reach out to people in other teams, other units, and other organizations and create those positive connections as well.

—*James W. Begun, PhD,*
James A. Hamilton Professor of Healthcare Management,
School of Public Health, University of Minnesota,
Minneapolis

ALL TOO OFTEN, we come home at the end of a long and stressful day, and the evening's dinner table conversation focuses on all the things that went wrong. We hone in on the negative without considering all the positive things that happened—the day's bright spots, the things that went well, and the people who brought us happiness. Taking a step back to understand the concept of mindfulness—a catchall term that basically means focusing on what *really* matters—encourages an inward approach as we make sense of the world around us. Adopting appreciative practice is a route to mindfulness—and a very real pathway to positivity.

Some hospital administrators begin their one-on-one and group meetings with a question: "Can you think of something that has happened since our last meeting that makes you proud?" Early on, the exercise might feel awkward because staff are not accustomed to this celebratory opener. Some people might not want to self-identify points of pride because it seems like bragging. Others might simply be embarrassed to be put on the spot. But if staff are given the opportunity to share what has made them proud, even if some opt to remain silent, the tradition often becomes everyone's favorite part of the meeting. Appreciative practice may be an individual choice—a tactic you can use at the meetings you run—or it may be an integral part of an organization's culture.

Research has repeatedly established a link between healthcare workers' mindful practices and their ability to provide competent, compassionate patient care. Tend the caregiver, it's said, and you ultimately tend the patient, too. Appreciative practice works in much the same way. If you practice positivity, you grease your cognitive circuitry in that area, making it an easier, more familiar technique to which you'll return. However brief those shared moments of pride are in the overall context of your hour- or two-hour-long meeting, appreciative practice helps you to begin on an up beat, to be present and attentive, and to connect with others in addition to strengthening those positive neurological circuits in your brain.

Appreciative practice begins by asking those present, "What is going well? For what or whom are you grateful?" At times, allowing moments of silence between each staffer's reflection is useful because it focuses on the positive and enables you and your team to adopt a more mindful approach. Permit time for everyone to speak if they'd like, and respectfully support those who wish to pass. As goofy as it might feel initially, it's a great way to start meetings. Even the hardest-hearted naysayer will be a believer before long.

Appreciative practice works by yourself, too. Good ways to begin your own personal appreciative practice might be to ask yourself the following questions:

- Whom do I appreciate today?
- For whom am I grateful, and why?
- Who are the organization's unsung heroes, the inconspicuous ones who work competently and diligently behind the scenes?
- How can I be wholly present, fully devoting my attention to the people in front of me? How can I connect with the person and not just the person's role, job, or purpose in the organization?

Your own appreciative practice might cultivate habits such as the following:

- **Sending personal notes or verbally expressing appreciation to people.** An expression of thanks might take the form of a brief e-mail, a handwritten note left on a desk, or a direct comment. The important thing is to do it, and to make such recognitions a habit.
- **Keeping a gratitude journal.** Jot down thoughts about those you're grateful for and why, or simply list, for each day, what rises to the top.
- **Scheduling regular alone time for yourself to reflect on what you are grateful for.** Whether you set aside 15–30 minutes in the morning to watch the sun rise while sipping your coffee or you turn off the radio on the way to work, make it a priority to channel your thoughts toward gratitude.
- **Improving your listening skills.** Good leaders listen first. Be present, and offer your full, unfettered attention

to the person who is speaking. When they have finished speaking, repeat what they said back to them, and then thoughtfully reply.

EXERCISE 1

Identify three to five of the most important "turning points" in your career that have led you to where you are now—serendipitous moments or opportunities that turned your career in a different direction. Reflect on these turning points and write about them in your journal.

EXERCISE 2

Make it a habit to start each meeting with an appreciative check-in. Ask, "What are you proud of since we last met? What is going well? Whom or what do you appreciate?"

RESOURCES

May, N., D. Becker, R. Frankel, J. Haizlip, R. Harmon, M. Plews-Ogan, J. Schorling, A. Williams, and D. Whitney. 2012. *Appreciative Inquiry in Healthcare*. Brunswick, OH: Crown Custom Publishing.

University of Virginia School of Medicine Center for Appreciative Practice. 2014. "Tools." Accessed November 11. www.medicine.virginia.edu/community-service/more /appreciative-practice/resources/appreciative-practices.

Define and Recalibrate Expectations

Have big vision, and set your expectations so that possibilities will emerge. Hire people who have a track record of high performance, coach them for confidence in owning their piece of the vision, and reward them when they accomplish results. People will take risks to achieve ever-higher results if they have permission to fail, and chances are greater that they will succeed!

—*Javier Hernandez-Lichtl, FACHE,*
CEO and corporate chief academic officer,
West Kendall Baptist Hospital—Baptist Health South Florida,
Miami

An *EXPECTATION* is commonly defined as a belief that something will or is likely to happen. You expect the sun to rise. You expect children to grow. You expect your paycheck to arrive.

But in business, including healthcare, expectations are much more than passive observations about the world, or things that simply happen with the passage of time. And being passive about your own expectations—thinking "Whatever will be, will be," for example—is a sure route to lukewarm leadership and tepid success.

Having expectations—and developing, refining, and recalibrating them—is an active, engaged process. All healthcare executives should set expectations for themselves and then actually believe they will happen. If you believe something will happen, you take positive steps in that direction. The most successful executives know and understand the power of positive thinking.

Have you ever found yourself accommodating a drop in your own personal standards in the name of getting things done? Perhaps you were part of a work group that had poor leadership or were a member of a losing team. As the group's expectations flag, individual members naturally experience a similar drop in their standards.

Here is where true leaders can set themselves apart. If you observe or feel an expectation slipping, you must stop the slide. Reestablish what your goals and standards are and where you're headed. You may even need to separate yourself from others who exert a negative influence on you. If possible, always ally yourself with teammates and mentors who have a positive outlook and similarly high expectations. That way, you know you'll be in sync.

A good way to hone your expectations is to ask yourself a few questions:

- What would I like to see happen?
- How can I positively affect outcomes?
- Who will be my best allies?
- When should work begin?
- What are the first steps I need to take to ensure a good result?

It goes without saying that to achieve your expectations, you should always offer your very best work. But how, exactly, do you do your best? One way is to seek out good mentors and model your behavior and strategies on theirs. Another is to study successful people: Find out who has achieved success in your industry, and examine the way they've approached problems, large or small. See if you can figure out the ingredients to their success.

As a leader, however, you will discover that not everyone will agree with your approach or share your motivation and savvy. Many brilliant, motivated people fail miserably as leaders because they lack the ability to motivate others. Great leaders understand that different people have different gifts, and they manage to assemble teams that maximize each member's strengths to contribute most effectively. Great leaders meet people, accept who they are, and draw out the best in each one.

Constantly set "stretch" goals: Challenge yourself to do and be better. Above all, hone in on goals that are in alignment with those of your organization and, when tackling them, maintain high expectations all the while. People like to be a part of an organization that feels visionary and a place that thinks beyond the ordinary. So, have those lofty personal expectations, and share your views about why and how great things can—and will—happen as you work with your colleagues.

Of course, big, meaty efforts take time and energy. They require attention, too. Be practical enough to try to complete the work that is important each day. And do not delay. Although your work shouldn't consist only of easy tasks or projects born of half-baked ideas, focusing your efforts on what *can* be done today will yield dividends tomorrow and in the weeks and years to come. Accomplishments have a way of naturally multiplying, especially under the pleasing glow of success.

EXERCISE 1

List five things critical to your organization's success, and then write down how those issues will look ten years down the road. Ask yourself the following questions:

- What would I like to see happen?
- How can I positively affect outcomes?
- What are the first steps to take to ensure a positive outcome?
- Who are the best people to help achieve this outcome?
- When should work begin?

EXERCISE 2

Pick a goal—personal or professional—that you have dreamed about but never really tried to accomplish. Write it down. Define the goal, and begin taking the first steps to accomplish it. Break it down into weekly action points, and check your progress each week.

RESOURCE

Manzoni, J.-F., and J.-L. Barsoux. 1998. "The Set-Up-To-Fail Syndrome." *Harvard Business Review* 76 (2): 101–13.

Be Interested in Others

As a healthcare executive early in your career, you will learn just how little you can accomplish alone. The sooner you learn this humbling lesson, the better. Creating meaningful relationships within your organization should be a top priority. These relationships will be the key to organizing and motivating your team to accomplish your organization's goals.

—*Zach McCluskey, MHA, RN, FACHE, CEO, HCA Parham Doctors' Hospital, Richmond, Virginia*

HEALTHCARE MANAGEMENT IS more than a job; it's a true calling. Few other vocations exist that so directly affect communities and people. And because healthcare is a highly regarded, noble field, healthcare executives occupy a privileged position at the helm. The very best healthcare executives feel an intense responsibility to really learn about their community's needs and then guide their organization to respond to those needs. But this is a tall order, and only the very best succeed.

With the introduction of endless sorts of technological gizmos, however—not to mention our modern predilection to share overly intimate details on the Internet and to spend every otherwise unoccupied moment fiddling with electronic devices—a new, unhealthy era of intense self-focus has arisen. Our collective attention span has atrophied. Coupled with the nation's growing self-absorption, the notions that "Everyone deserves a prize" and "No one should be singled out for special treatment" have yielded a common and sometimes overwhelming sense of entitlement. "You can do or be anything you want" and "The sky's the limit" are frequent words of encouragement. Although these sentiments may be true, no one who's truly successful got anywhere without a lot of hard work, determination, and the steadfast support of other people along the way.

In your role as a healthcare manager, you're in the cheering section, behind the concession stand, in the dugout with the clipboard—but not on the playing field. You exist to support others and organize systems so that, together, they can provide patients with the best possible care. In that capacity, it's imperative that you exhibit—and actually possess—a keen interest in others, not that you just be an interesting person yourself. Ask questions of others. Be curious about your colleagues' backstories—where they grew up, what their jobs are, and what their career trajectories have been. When others talk, receive what they say: Be present, listen, observe, intuit—and *remember*.

Some healthcare administration students complete residencies and, as part of that, prepare an administrative residency plan at the outset. The purpose of this exercise is to derive learning objectives to help the student understand the wide variety of roles in the healthcare organization. Some students might rotate through various departments, as medical and nursing students do, to get a feel for the breadth of work roles throughout the organization. Devoting a week or two to each department—from housekeeping to IT, from surgery to transplants—can be a great way to gather perspective. Taking half-hour tours and shaking hands with a few people, on the other hand, just isn't going to cut it.

If you have the chance to rotate through different departments in your organization, ask questions of (and really listen to) those you meet. Find out what problems they face, what frustrations they experience, what disruptions and inefficiencies they deal with, and what ideas they have to make the place run more smoothly. Get to know these colleagues as people. Build relationships as best you can, finding out what it takes to clean and prep a room for a new patient, to navigate and organize insurance paperwork, to answer phones, to be in charge of a unit's nurses, and to keep the parking garage and grounds clean and neat. Understand what issues frontline workers encounter each day. Knowing what they do is a great way to be an authentic, effective leader.

Here are some tips for being interested in others and focusing less on yourself:

- **Learn to ask questions, and listen carefully and thoughtfully to the responses.** Ask people what's difficult about their jobs as well as what they find most rewarding. What processes and systems are ineffective or inefficient? What ideas do they have for improvements? Ask people what they care most about and what they find personally rewarding outside of work. Make sure you don't interrupt them while they're talking or turn the focus back on yourself.

- **When someone pays you a compliment, pay it backward.** After you say thank you, acknowledge that you had a lot of good help from many people along the way. Show that you're the kind of person who offers compliments and praise with regularity and ease, someone who recognizes that little is accomplished without the wisdom and help of others.

- **Replace fears about how you are being perceived with curiosity about others.** People often express worry about how they came across in an interview or while giving a presentation. Swap such thoughts with a determination to be inquisitive about others. If you are interested in others, there is no room left for you to worry about yourself.

- **Don't judge or get personal.** You will meet plenty of people who hold different political views, religious beliefs, and values than you do. Your job is not to judge or disapprove of others (unless their preferences and beliefs cause hostility, poor job performance, or fractiousness within your organization) but to be curious and interested in them as people. You are not out to preach or convert.

- **Celebrate important occasions.** Keep a master list of birthdays, and be diligent about sending cards or e-mails to staff wishing them well. Beyond birthdays, send notes of congratulations to colleagues who have received an honor or who have excelled at something.

- **Write thank-you notes.** This one is important. In an era rife with technology, there is no replacement for a handwritten note of thanks. Keep a stash of basic thank-you notes in your desk or home office. If someone invites you to a social event, gives you a gift, or does something that deserves a special thank-you, send them a note of gratitude within 48 hours. If you're not able to handwrite the note, e-mail is the second-best option.

- **Exchange the pronouns *I, me,* and *my* with *we, us,* and *our*.** This puts the focus on teamwork and reinforces the group's efforts.

- **Keep your opinions to yourself unless it's related to the task at hand.** When asked for your opinion, frame it as something that "we should" do. That way, it seems less like an opinion and more like an accepted fact.

- **Learn and remember others' names.** Make it a habit. In meetings, if you don't know everyone sitting around the table, ask someone to help you with their names and positions, and write them down. Before meeting with people you have not met, look them up online and become familiar with their background.

It is said that true character is the way you treat those who can do nothing for you. When you are truly interested in others without regard for what they can offer you, you will possess the foundation on which others' trust is built. Trust is necessary for honest and transparent communication, and many people can smell feigned interest from miles away. Always approach others as people with amazing stories rather than as people who are merely a work title or an organizational role to you.

EXERCISE 1

Complete an emotional and social intelligence survey instrument to identify areas for development. (One such instrument is the Hay Group's Emotional and Social Competency Inventory Survey, available at www.haygroup.com/leadershipandtalenton demand/ourproducts/item_details.aspx?itemid=58&type=3&t=2.)

EXERCISE 2

After identifying development areas in Exercise 1, attend a workshop, read books, ask your mentor for advice, and practice unlearning old habits and relearning new ones.

EXERCISE 3

Make it a habit to learn and remember names. When making rounds, learn at least one new name every time. Associate the person's name with a mnemonic.

RESOURCES

Forni, P. M. 2002. *Choosing Civility: The Twenty-Five Rules of Considerate Conduct.* New York: St. Martin's Press.

Goleman, D., R. Boyatzis, and A. McKee. 2013. *Primal Leadership: Unleashing the Power of Emotional Intelligence.* Cambridge, MA: Harvard Business Review Press.

Use Mobile Devices and Social Media Wisely

Leveraging social networks provides a real opportunity to use your voice, build online visibility, and connect with others who share similar interests. These connections can help build your professional network, but it is essential that you actively manage your online reputation. Exercise good judgment, and keep confidential, private, sensitive, and proprietary business and patient information far, far away from social media.

—Christina Beach Thielst, FACHE,
health administration and governance consultant,
Santa Barbara, California

STROLL ACROSS ANY university campus and you'll see students walking like zombies, texting or chatting on their cell phones, oblivious to the world around them. Such is our technological age—one of insularity riddled with self-absorption and a level of "connectivity" that actually breeds disconnect and discontent. Our devotion to devices and social media offers a cautionary tale because this technology has in fact become hazardous to the health of conversation and interpersonal, face-to-face communication. And in healthcare, as in other businesses, it's how you communicate person-to-person that *really* matters.

Technology's big sell was the time savings it was supposed to provide. However, when used unwisely, these devices and platforms are actually time thieves. Sites such as Facebook, Twitter, Google+, Pinterest, and other social channels consume vast amounts of time and energy that could be spent more productively. Even highly regarded networking sites such as LinkedIn, which can facilitate professional connections and collaborations, can suck you in if you spend too much time cultivating online relationships. The key is leveraging technology and social sites in moderation and knowing when to get out from behind your desk and away from your computer screen into the real world of real-time human interaction—not screen-to-screen but *in the flesh*.

Social media sites tempt people to cultivate robust online presences and to post information, pictures, and details about their personal lives that they might not otherwise offer in person—sometimes even the kind of information that may damage their professional image and reputation. Some sites provide electronic diaries that may seem private but are accessible to nearly anyone; even the comments you post on just about any website can be tracked back to you.

You should understand the risks associated with these sorts of activities so that you don't do something careless that can have lasting consequences. When you're searching for a job, you should know exactly what exists about you online, and if you don't like what you see, do something about it before it becomes a problem for you. Honestly, the best strategy to scrub your online image is to be sure it's squeaky clean from the get-go.

Some might perceive social networking as professionally advantageous because it enables you to tap colleagues on a more personal basis. So what's the difference between social and professional networking? The dividing line is blurry. But it's important to keep your private and work lives distinct.

Like social media sites, the omnipresence of devices also seems to exert a gravitational pull toward networking. Smartphones and other mobile devices have become a necessity for many of us, but sometimes it's wholly inappropriate to pull your phone out to check a message, answer a call, or see what your friends are up to on Instagram. Know when it's OK to use your device—and when it's not OK.

Here are some Device 101 pointers to consider:

- **Turn off your phone during meetings, and stow it.** Unless you're expecting an urgent call, keep your phone out of sight so you're not tempted to glance at it. Give the meeting and your colleagues the full attention they deserve.
- **Checking messages during a meeting is rude and inappropriate.** No looking at messages, no typing, no texting—nothing. Don't do it.
- **If you must take a call, ask to be excused and step out of the room.** Begin your conversation once you've fully exited, not when you're halfway to the door. Keep it short and get back to the task at hand.
- **Many states have outlawed texting while driving; do nothing but drive when behind the wheel of your car.** Messages can wait until you're home or in the office. If you do your very best thinking in the car, get a digital recorder to record your ideas or use a phone equipped with a recorder to take hands-free notes.

And here are some social media considerations:

- **If you're a blogger or social media user, make sure your entries don't contain anything dicey.** The same goes for any photos you post of your activities. Would you blush if your mom read or saw them? What about your colleagues? Would you mind if those pictures you posted were on the front page of the newspaper?
- **If you decide to use social media, take a close look at your profile.** Does it reflect what you want business contacts or prospective employers to see?

- **Feel free to post content about your job search, career, or professional interests.** Be frank about what you're looking for and what you're interested in, and "like" professional groups or organizations that are in your career domain. If you participate in online discussions about professional topics, keep your comments clean and concise. No crazy rants, flip language, or questionable references.
- **Take a close look at the friends and groups you're connected with on social media.** Do they project the type of image you desire? Choose your friends wisely.
- **Never post someone else's image or information unless you have explicit permission to do so.** Otherwise, you could be held civilly or criminally liable. Also, never post information or photos that would violate your organization's network use policy or HIPAA (Health Insurance Portability and Accountability Act) privacy rules.
- **Never use your employer's logo on your personal site without permission.** If you share your views online, do so only as an individual, not as a representative of your organization. If you feel angry or passionate about a subject, wait until you're calm and clear headed before posting a reaction or statement.
- **If you're posting on a website, do so on your own time and device.** Respect your employer's time and property—don't use work time and equipment to participate in social media or online discussions.
- **Think before you post.** Nothing online is ever truly private.

As with diet, exercise, alcohol, and most of life, moderation is key when it comes to technology and social media. Know when to use your devices and for what reasons. Excellent, high-quality work still stems from clear-minded individuals who are able to process without distraction—and smartphones, Snapchat, and Instagram have nothing to do with it.

Many have learned hard, career-ending lessons when they've not tamed their online habits. So remember: If you do use a social or professional networking site, make sure it reflects your personal brand. Use it to highlight your education, experience, skills, and professional and community service. Let it show you as a thoughtful, perceptive human being. There isn't a lot of room for error, so it's best to be careful.

EXERCISE 1

Google yourself and see what comes up. Note what you were surprised by and what you'd have preferred to see at the top of the search results.

EXERCISE 2

Review your profiles on social media websites to be sure they reflect your personal brand. Ask an expert for advice.

RESOURCES

Thielst, C. B. 2014. *Applying Social Media Technologies in Healthcare Environments.* Chicago: Healthcare Information and Management Systems Society.

————. 2013. *Social Media in Healthcare: Connect, Communicate, Collaborate,* second edition. Chicago: Health Administration Press.

Harness the Power
of Mindfulness

Inviting stillness, inquiry, and reflection. Paying attention in the
moment and not glancing at our iPhones every minute.
Breathing. Offering ourselves and others the gift of a loving-
kindness meditation. Pausing before responding in order to
be generous and kind in comments to colleagues, students,
and everyone we greet each day. All of this is what mindfulness
offers me as a leader. We are creating a new generation of
leaders in healthcare by offering these ideas and concepts to
our students, faculty, and healthcare providers at UVA.

—*Dorrie K. Fontaine, RN, PhD, FAAN,*
dean and Sadie Heath Cabaniss Professor of Nursing,
School of Nursing, University of Virginia,
Charlottesville

"ATTENTION," WROTE PHILOSOPHER Simone Weil, "is the
rarest and purest form of generosity." But while the concept is
simple enough, being *truly* present is incredibly hard to do. Our
attentiveness is continually interrupted by a host of forces, especially electronic ones, that rob us from the moment. And although
many routinely blame their gizmos, the real culprit is Americans'
propensity to live either in the past or the future—not the present.
We, and those around us—from our children to our spouses, from
our colleagues to our clients—suffer as a result.

The most authentic leaders understand what it means to pay homage to the present. They practice paying attention and consciously notice new things—those with whom they come into contact, the connections that exist between others, the impact of the environment, how their bodies respond to particular situations, and how their minds interpret external stimuli. This practice, in its essence, is mindfulness—and it has the ability to shape one's destiny in powerful ways. Research has revealed that, if practiced effectively and often, mindfulness exerts a positive effect on health and well-being by redirecting stress and anxiety. Research has also shown that those who practice mindfulness are often more charismatic, are more creative and innovative, are less judgmental, and tend to procrastinate less often. Being mindful, not "mind-full," is simply a better way to live, to work, and to care.

Though a certain amount of life and work involves routine and repetition, *all* activities can be conducted mindfully. If you operate continually (or even partially) on autopilot, you might miss something important—a nuance, a random but inspired idea or notion, or perhaps a connection to another that may lead to a better practice, a different way of thinking, perhaps even a new job. It pays to pay attention.

When you live mindfully, serendipity often follows. Matt, for example, told his former professor and adviser how frustrated and restless he was at his current job, mentioning that he wanted to return to an urban area in the Mid-Atlantic. His professor kept Matt's card, mulled over possibilities for him, and a few weeks later found himself seated next to the CEO of a Richmond hospital who asked him whether he knew of any good candidates for a certain job she needed to fill. The professor gave her Matt's card, and although Matt did not get that particular job, he did land another position at the Richmond hospital a few months later. Invariably, connections are made if people are open to them. In Matt's case, a positive outcome resulted from paying attention, making connections, getting the right people together, and being open to serendipity.

Mindfulness can also be practiced in more deliberate, less serendipitous ways. Some hospitals teach clinicians activities such as the relaxation response—a 20-minute breathing and visualization exercise that involves a pattern of head-to-toe muscle tension and release—as a way to deal with stress and anxiety. Other hospitals offer regular meditation and yoga classes or have a special quiet room where clinicians and others can go to recalibrate after difficult interactions or emotional cases. Some hospital staff deliberately re-center themselves in a collective pause amid the chaos of an emergency department; others observe a moment of silence after a patient's death or after the stress of sharing a bad diagnosis. However mindfulness manifests itself in a healthcare organization, those *at all levels* of the organization must be able to tap their inner resources. If the organization does not emphasize and provide access to such mindful practices and behavior, burnout and turnover—which are costly in terms of both financial and psychological bottom lines—often ensue. Healthcare is a rewarding field precisely because the work done matters so much. If healthcare workers have no way to keep their spirits buoyant and to deal effectively with adversity, their tenure will be short, and ultimately their impact will be diminished.

There are many ways to practice mindfulness, but all have in common a movement toward relaxation and a conscious effort to center on the present without distraction. In your practice, do what works best for you. Discipline and a certain suspension of disbelief may be required, but the rewards are many. The following are a few techniques that are used for mindfulness:

- Meditation
- Centering prayer
- Yoga
- Exercise
- Writing
- A mental focus on a certain visual, such as mountains or a body of water

Whichever technique proves best, make it a habit. Put it on your schedule. Some hospital CEOs meditate with colleagues each week before breakfast. Others wake up at 5 a.m. and spend time writing in their journals. Still others take a solitary jog on deserted streets at sunrise. The point is to do it regularly. And keep in mind that mindfulness isn't about checking something off a list; it's about making room to breathe and taking time to be still and present—nothing more. You don't have to become a New Age guru to do it—just a thoughtful person aiming to continue to be more so.

What can you do to be more mindful at work? Ellen Langer, who has studied mindfulness for 40 years, offers the following advice:

- As you determine your level of emotional investment in a problem, ask yourself, "Is this a tragedy or merely an inconvenience?"
- Imagine that your thoughts are totally transparent and visible to those around you.
- Think about how best to integrate work and life, not balance the two in equal parts.
- Familiarize yourself with an issue's "other side" to understand that both sides have good arguments.
- Seek win–win solutions.
- Show compassion to others when they may not be in a mindful place; aim to understand where they are coming from.
- When giving feedback to employees or evaluating their performance, be sure to emphasize that it is *your* perspective and not a universal one. Be willing to be wrong and to change your views when you receive additional information.
- Don't rely solely on checklists or computer-prompted questions that lack a qualitative component; they encourage mindlessness.

EXERCISE 1

Read more about mindfulness by selecting one of the recommended resources, or Google the word *mindfulness*.

EXERCISE 2

Make a list of three mindful techniques, and schedule 20 minutes on three different mornings in a given week to try each. Then select the technique that works for you.

RESOURCES

Benson, H., and M. Z. Klipper. 2000. *The Relaxation Response.* New York: HarperCollins.

Bourgeault, C. 2004. *Centering Prayer and Inner Awakening.* Lanham, MD: Cowley Publications.

Kabat-Zinn, J. 2005. *Coming to Our Senses: Healing Ourselves and the World Through Mindfulness.* New York: Hyperion.

Langer, E. 2014. "Mindfulness in the Age of Complexity." *Harvard Business Review* 91 (3): 68–73.

Marturano, J. 2014. *Finding the Space to Lead: A Practical Guide to Mindful Leadership.* New York: Bloomsbury Press.

Salzberg, S. 2013. *Real Happiness at Work: Meditations for Accomplishment, Achievement, and Peace.* New York: Workman Publishing Company.

Develop a Personal Brand

> Early in my career, I was described in an annual review as "non-threateningly aggressive"—and while I'm not sure I appreciated at the time what this meant, today it's become abundantly clear. Now, as I work with and hire others, the importance of being able to get a job done cannot be overstated. For employees, this translates into being tenacious, following up without being too pushy or demonstrating a lack of respect. It's no longer enough to simply complete a task or assignment; you must get good work done well, and on time, while demonstrating respect for and grace toward those around you. If you show these attributes, you'll be rewarded throughout your career with opportunities that are both challenging and fulfilling.
>
> —*Tiffany P. Lange, president,*
> *Lange Consulting LLC,*
> *Richmond, Virginia*

As CHILDREN AND adolescents, we learned ways to fit in by having the latest clothes, bicycles, handbags, cars, hairstyles, electronic gadgets, or club memberships—tangibles that often felt like the sole pathway to status and acceptance. At these early points in life, being different felt like a deficit. What you realize as a grownup, however, is that standing out—and standing brave in your skin, with your values and morals intact—has power, merit, and immense worth. Being wholly yourself is always better than trying to follow pathways determined by others; the best executives stand tall as who they are.

The transition from lemming to leader happens rather suddenly. When you enter the professional world, it becomes important to show how you're different from the pack. How you stand out and what values you bring and add to a place become your personal brand. These traits are critical to your success in any organization, healthcare included—and they have little to do with clothes, cars, or memberships and everything to do with who you really are and the singular assets, skills, and values you bring.

As children, we're taught a set of values and behaviors that reflect those values. And while not everyone receives the same set of instructions at the outset, by the time one moves into a position of managerial responsibility, knowing basic manners is essential. There is real economic value in cultivating your personal brand, so be sure you have the basics of politeness and good manners thoroughly covered.

Executive skills classes are traditionally part of every healthcare administration graduate student's coursework, and they are particularly helpful to those who need to polish their manners to ensure a smooth transition into the workplace. It goes without saying that first impressions usually stick and that negative first impressions are nearly impossible to overturn. Many students and job seekers never quite recover from interview gaffes committed through lack of basic manners and social mores. Don't be one of them.

Managing what impression you make on others is a big part of working in any profession, and such impression management goes beyond your emotional and social intelligence. *How* you show the tenets of your personal code—your behaviors, actions, and responses—matters immensely. To have a successful personal brand you must first be open to seeing yourself wholly and critically, so monitor yourself and others' reactions to you closely, and ask for feedback. The best way to know how others perceive you is to undergo a 360-degree performance evaluation, which involves input from your managers, peers, subordinates, and others.

But you don't have to wait for others to tell you what personal gaps and skill deficits you have. You can buoy the impression you make by absorbing lessons on business etiquette from books, by noticing how people you admire as professionals manage impressions, and by asking others what they think are important attributes of leaders.

Here are a few key ingredients to inform your personal brand:

- **Know the rules of civility.** Start with a book on business etiquette to ensure you're current. In our increasingly multicultural society, understanding appropriate manners for international settings is also important. Social and business customs in one country may be different in another. Be sure you know the rules *before* you go abroad or interact with someone visiting from another country.

- **Get along.** Embrace feedback and criticism, and acknowledge and appreciate differences. Understand that you don't have to like everyone you work with, but you do have to get along. Assume that others have positive intentions, and always remember to be humble and nice and to abandon any sense of entitlement. If you have an attitude, lose it.

- **Honor professional relationships.** Relationships take time to develop, so don't become too familiar with others in your work or profession when you first get to know them—particularly if they occupy a position of authority. Professional relationships may overlap with personal and social relationships, but not necessarily. Some people choose to keep their work relationships strictly professional, and you must respect that choice. Proceed here with caution and care.

- **Be trustworthy.** If someone tells you something in confidence, always keep that confidence. You'll cause irreparable harm to your credibility if you're deemed untrustworthy (and it only takes one mistake for this to happen).

- **Be grateful.** People rarely find success in isolation. When someone pays you a compliment or gives you recognition, first say thank you, then share the praise by pointing to others' role in your success. If a colleague agrees to serve as a reference, send a thank-you note. Remember, too, that if you do something careless or stupid, it will reflect poorly on others who have vouched for you—an incentive to always do your best.

- **Run good meetings.** Have a purpose. Develop an agenda, and stick to it. Identify action items and items that are for information only. Agree on standards of behavior and process, and know how to disagree with others respectfully. If you're attending another's meeting, turn off your mobile device and be present. Even if you're not feeling fully engaged, fake it as best you can because people will notice your demeanor. Be on time, and if you have to miss the meeting, be thoughtful enough to let the organizer know in advance.

- **Be engaged and engaging.** *Really* listen to what others are saying, and attempt to understand their reasons. Take in body language to gauge how the conversation is going. Consider what the other person wants. And be an optimist: Remind others that you're seeking a positive outcome.

- **Learn.** Aim to broaden your horizons, and be willing to start on the ground floor to build a career. Be curious, and take an interest in what others do. Don't ever be too good for a task—everyone has to start somewhere.

Keep these ideas in mind, too:

- A first-class education or Ivy-league affiliation doesn't entitle you to a good job or give you a particular advantage if you do get one.

- Being smart in school doesn't mean you're smart at everything. Listen, and show you can learn from others.
- Working hard doesn't mean you deserve an A or a pay raise.
- Just because someone is nice doesn't mean they will or should make exceptions to their standards or rules in your case.
- Just because you've always been at the top of your class doesn't mean you'll be the top performer in a professional setting. Learning business takes time; employers care less about whether you know how to write a business plan and more about whether you'll be able to execute it.
- Don't plagiarize. Just because information is freely available online doesn't mean it's yours for the taking and doesn't require citation.
- Just because you're addicted to your mobile device doesn't mean you should attend to it in the company of others. Doing so suggests you're insensitive and immature and gives the impression that your phone is more important than what—or who—is right in front of you.
- Just because you or your parents know someone socially doesn't mean that person owes you favors or special treatment.

So what works?

- Treat all people with kindness and respect, not just those who can be of use to you.
- Know your values and the behaviors consistent with those values.
- Don't take yourself too seriously. Be self-deprecating so that others know you don't always have to be right—and they don't think you can't relax.

- Learn and practice mindfulness (see Lesson 8). Be in the moment. Good things happen when you pay attention.
- Set your own boundaries, and respect those of others.
- Improve your grammar, use proper English, avoid slang and profanity, and drop college speak such as *dude, like, you know, totally, awesome,* and *no problem* from your vocabulary.
- Don't drink (or drink only in moderation) at business functions, whatever the function and regardless of what others are doing. Never have more than two alcoholic drinks at any business function.
- When someone asks you a question, don't respond by saying they've asked a good question. If you need to buy time, a moment of silence before responding shows you're being thoughtful.
- Remember and use the following words liberally:
  - Please
  - Thank you
  - You're welcome
  - I was wrong
  - I'm sorry
  - What do you think?
- When you commit to follow up or to meet a deadline, do it. Being too busy is not an acceptable excuse.
- Excuses aren't the same as apologies. Don't say why you didn't get something done or made a mistake; say you're sorry and it won't happen again—then follow through.
- Avoid speaking ill of anyone behind their back, even if they deserve it.
- Learn the expected behaviors in a healthy work environment (see Lesson 36).
- Don't lose your temper. If you're about to, take a break.

- Be nice to everyone, and remember that anyone in the organization can be influential. It is not about the title.

EXERCISE 1

List three of your best traits, and try writing a one-sentence tagline that expresses your personal brand.

EXERCISE 2

Complete a Johari Window exercise (http://kevan.org/johari) to understand how others see you compared to how you see yourself.

RESOURCES

Pachter, B. 2013. *The Essentials of Business Etiquette: How to Greet, Eat, and Tweet Your Way to Success.* New York: McGraw-Hill.

Post, P., and P. Post. 2005. *Emily Post's The Etiquette Advantage in Business: Personal Skills for Professional Success,* second edition. New York: William Morrow.

Write Well

Written words hold tremendous power: power to encourage, to inspire, to criticize, to tear down, to educate, to coerce, and to create. More than spoken words, it's those that are written—whether they're carved in stone, scribbled on a piece of paper, or typed on a computer screen—that carry a sense of permanence as they're rapidly disseminated, saved for future reference, and repeatedly read. Written words can sometimes reach a vast audience and, for that reason, must be carefully wrought with the understanding of their lasting impact.

Effective writing is invaluable and uncommon and must not be confined solely to formal papers or letters. It's a habit that requires dedication, development, and consistent practice, however, beginning with the simple notes and written messages we daily share with one another. Make a habit of writing well beginning today.

—Patrick D. Shay, PhD, assistant professor, Department of Health Care Administration, Trinity University, San Antonio, Texas

SOME SAY WRITTEN communication is fading into oblivion. Today, e-mail and text messages—which often don't employ proper grammar and draw on a whole lexicon of abbreviations—make up the bulk of social and business correspondence. These formats don't offer the benefits of the handwritten note or formal business letter, however; nor have they adequately replaced it.

To write well, you have to know more than good grammar and punctuation. And whereas college courses required papers of a minimum length that rewarded wordiness, the business world demands the opposite. That one-page executive summary you're writing must elegantly contain all the contents of a ten-page essay. Executives have neither the time nor the attention span to read lengthy missives. They want to glean the main points and the recommended next steps. The art of concise writing is tricky and is only achieved through practice.

But whittled-down, tight language doesn't mean your writing has to be bland. Activate your words by avoiding forms of the verb *to be*. Use action words to convey meaning, and consider the effect of powerful adjectives. Use contractions to avoid robot-speak. Intersperse long sentences with short ones. Use bullets to break up long passages of text. And keep the tone as conversational as you can.

Following are some tips for specific types of business communications.

EXECUTIVE SUMMARIES

Think of an executive summary as your elevator speech: You've got 90 to 120 seconds to convey your idea and no more. Be succinct and engaging. Boil it down to three to five main points. Use language that is easy to grasp without being too elementary. Don't obfuscate with fancy verbiage.

Note the difference between these two examples:

> **Version 1:** Our internal quality improvement team is reading case studies. The studies are of three similar companies in the Mid-Atlantic with roughly equivalent numbers of patients, physicians, and nurses and operating budgets of at least $350 million annually. These medical centers are nationally ranked and have Magnet designation. With this research and by following

their examples, we will figure out how to be a better, stronger, more profitable company.

Version 2: Case studies of similar institutions will help us chart a path toward Magnet designation and profitability. The best institutions have

- a profound emphasis on patients,
- an exceptional devotion to safety and quality, and
- a focus on caregivers' compassion, resilience, and satisfaction.

BUSINESS CORRESPONDENCE, THANK-YOU NOTES, AND INTERNAL MEMOS

All thank-you notes should be sent and postmarked within 48 hours of the interview (or hosted meal, reference provided, professional favor, or other courtesy). Use a stamp rather than putting it through your organization's postal meter (keep some stamps in your desk drawer).

If an administrative professional assists you with your correspondence, proofread all letters before signing. A business letter should be like a framed piece of art: unmarred, centered, straight, on quality letterhead, and of course with no errors in grammar or punctuation. When the letter is folded into a business envelope, make creases straight and sharp. The addressee's name, title, and address should be correctly spelled—no exceptions. If you receive someone's business card, mimic exactly what's there.

Never use fancy fonts or paper that is anything other than strictly classic. Be consistent in using a standard typeface (e.g., Times New Roman, Arial) and font size (e.g., 12 point). Do not mix typefaces, and avoid excessive use of boldface, underlining, and italics. Don't rely solely on spell-checker because it can change proper names into incorrectly spelled ones. When you sign your name, do so in ink—in a contrasting color, if you can. A stamped or scanned signature implies you were uninvolved in the letter-writing process.

E-MAIL MESSAGES

Although e-mail has become the standard way to communicate at work, it can be inefficient and is prone to unintended misinterpretation. Before you hit "send," consider these factors:

- **Make sure that e-mail is the right communication tool for the job.** If you suspect that your e-mail will result in a lot of questions, a face-to-face meeting would be better. Know the difference.
- **Consider your e-mail as important as a written letter.** Just because it's an e-mail doesn't mean you should abandon capitalization, grammar, punctuation rules, and proper spacing. Don't type the content of your e-mail in the subject line as if it were a text message. Don't use texting abbreviations in an e-mail. Start your e-mail with a greeting, and close it with *Sincerely, Thank you, Do let me know,* or a similar phrase. Type your name at the end.
- **Get to the point.** Use the first three sentences to tell people what they need to know. If your colleagues are trying to schedule a meeting, don't go into detail about how busy you are—simply say when you're available.
- **One message, one topic.** Communicate in a straight line without going off on tangents or other topics that water down the main point.
- **Specify who should respond—and be clear about your deadline.** You can even note the deadline in the subject line, along with two to three words summarizing the topic.
- **Use common sense when forwarding e-mails.** Don't make your recipient wade through the e-mail muck of a forwarded string. Start fresh, offering a sentence or two of context. Also, make sure the message you're forwarding does not contain sensitive information or snarky remarks.

- **Be transparent and inclusive.** If you are writing an e-mail that affects more than one person, include everyone on the same e-mail, addressing it to those who are critically involved and copying those who are tangentially involved.
- **Simplify your e-mail signature.** Be sure your electronic "business card" is simple and straightforward and doesn't have your favorite quote, a lengthy description of your job title, and other redundant information.
- **Don't send anything you wouldn't want everyone in your company (or your mom) to read.** No office politics, snarky remarks, inappropriate forwards, or profanity.
- **No emoticons.** Not now, not ever. Don't do it.

There are also rules to follow when receiving e-mails. The following are the most important:

- **Don't make assumptions about the sender's emotional state.** Hurried messages may seem to have an emotional tone that was not intended. If you get such a message, pause. Switch tasks. Then reread the message later before you respond.
- **Don't reply to confrontational messages.** E-mail silence offers you a position of poise and, frankly, of power. Better to meet in person or discuss by phone.
- **Ask for clarification in person.** Seeking clarity in person or over the phone, rather than by another e-mail, will save you time in the long run.
- **Keep organized.** Use color coding and folders to organize e-mails relating to the same issue. Block spam and junk mail, but check those folders periodically to ensure colleagues and clients don't get caught in your filter.
- **Don't respond to every message right away.** Designate regular periods during your workday to read and respond to e-mails. If you get in the habit of answering

work-related e-mails during your off-hours or from home, your colleagues will expect that level of connectivity.

- **Set boundaries about personal e-mail.** Let your friends and family know when you check your personal e-mail. Set aside time to check and respond to e-mail before and after work hours.

EXERCISE 1

Write a one-page essay about any topic using no more than eight instances of the verb *to be*.

EXERCISE 2

Buy personalized note cards, and start practicing the art of writing notes.

RESOURCES

Connor, P. 2014. "Business Email." Colorado State University Writing@CSU. Accessed November 11. http://writing.colostate.edu/guides/documents/business_writing/business_email/index.cfm.

Mind Tools. 2014. "Communication Skills: Communicating in Writing." Accessed November 11. www.mindtools.com/page8.html#writing.

Silverman, D. 2009. "4 Tips for Writing Better Email." *Harvard Business Review* Blog Network. Posted March 6. http://blogs.harvardbusiness.org/silverman/2009/03/4-tips-for-better-business-wri.html.

Speak Well

Speaking in public is often seen as one of the most terror-inducing activities a person can imagine, but, like so many other things in life generally and management specifically, practice can overcome even the worst fears. The key is to engage your audience— no matter how large or how small, how public or how private— with your sincerity. After that, the speaking just flows.

—*Stephen S. Mick, PhD, FACHE,*
professor emeritus of health administration,
Virginia Commonwealth University, Richmond

SPEAKING WELL MEANS getting information across clearly, effectively, and—with luck—memorably. Those who speak well project confidence and authority. Whether you are addressing a group or speaking informally with someone one-on-one, *how* you speak says a lot about you.

Whatever the situation, here are some simple questions to keep in mind when you're speaking:

- **What is my aim?** Am I trying to inform, persuade, or both?
- **Who is in my audience?** How much do they know about my subject? Why would they be interested in or care about what I have to say? No one likes to listen to a speaker who talks down to the audience or speaks over their heads. If

you know your audience, you can direct the content of your message appropriately.

- **What are the main points I want to make?** Rather than send out a tidal wave of information, you should give audience members three to five takeaways. Tell them what those points are at the beginning, explain each one, and then remind them of the points at the end.

- **What's your call to action?** What do you want people to do after they listen to you? You must invite them to buy your idea, give you a job, join your club, or give you a raise. Don't assume they will infer—hypercommunicate (see Lesson 26).

Try to get a solid sense of the physical environment in which you'll be speaking well beforehand. Consider how large the room is, how large your audience will likely be, and what equipment (e.g., microphone, podium, lavalier that travels with you and projects your voice) will be necessary. Will you show slides on a screen? Will the audience have an opportunity to ask questions during or after your talk—and if so, how will they be heard? How long will your portion of the presentation last?

An oral presentation often follows a particular format, such as the following:

- **Start with an icebreaker.** This is your chance to harness the audience's attention. Good at jokes? Tell a funny story about yourself that segues into one of your main messages or themes. Other presenters ask for a show of hands in response to a particular question. The beginning is a critical time to introduce yourself—especially when speaking to large audiences—even if you believe you know everyone in the room. Explain what you do and why you're there.

- **Introduce and frame the topic.** Offer your audience a sense of how long you'll be talking, which will help keep their attention.
- **Announce your outline.** Inform the audience which three to five takeaway points you'll focus on.
- **Name and number your central points.** "Now let us move on to point number one. . . ."
- **Flesh out each point with a real-life story or data that succinctly illustrate its significance.** Then pause to let the point soak in. Beware of tossing in too many numbers, however; keep the data to a minimum and be sure they support your argument.
- **Break up your conclusion into four parts:** (1) Review what your main points were; (2) be clear what the takeaway or action plan is; (3) thank the audience for their time and attention; and (4) invite them to ask questions or make comments.

Inevitably, snags will arise before or during your presentation despite the best-laid plans—and, frankly, that's life. Your microphone may need a new battery or produce deafening interference or feedback, your slides may be out of focus, or your computer may crash. Your voice may give out. But as with everything in work and life, it's how you roll with it—and being able to do so, of course—that truly shows your mettle. *You* are the key ingredient in any presentation (the technology is, and should be, largely ancillary), so what *you* have to share and how *you* compel others is what's most important.

Keep in mind that how you handle complications says a lot about your leadership ability. If something goes awry, try to have a backup plan, and remain calm and good humored about whatever trouble has arisen. Never berate your support staff in front of others, whether verbally or with stares that kill. Even if you feel your stomach churning, your skin breaking out in perspiration, and your neck and face turning red and splotchy with embarrassment, do the best you can. Hold your head high and remember that you're on display. Do your best to act with confidence, even if you don't feel an inkling of it.

If problems arise, don't continually refer to them or apologize for them. If you truly need to stop your presentation to address an issue, make it an excuse for a ten-minute break for the audience to stretch their legs while you regroup. Don't make the audience sit there while you and your team try to fix what's broken. Move on as best you can.

Here are some tips for polishing your speech:

- **Never simply read what's on the screen.** Use bulleted note cards or cues instead. Your audience, unless they're in kindergarten, can already read.

- **Your gestures and posture should be natural and comfortable.** Stand firm on both feet, and avoid rocking, leaning, or slouching. If you're holding a microphone, know how far (usually six to eight inches) to hold it from your mouth.

- **Be aware of and avoid distracting behaviors.** Avoid jingling change in your pocket, touching your face, or playing with your hair.

- **Never curse.** Don't use even grade B swear words.

- **Be aware of not only what you say but *how* you say it.** This includes your volume, pitch, tone, stutter, and any stammering or use of filler words such as *like, you know,* and *um.* Finish sentences rather than stringing them together with *and* or *um.* When you speak, don't let your statements sound like questions by ending them with a rising pitch.

- **Evaluate your audience's response as you speak.** Watch for what they react to, and always make good eye contact.

- **Always, *always* rehearse.** Practice in front of a mirror, with a recording device, in front of an honest friend, or better yet, with a video camera. Self-evaluation is a powerful motivation for changing behaviors.

When you're speaking with difficult or rude people—or with those who interrupt—always remember that you can't go wrong with listening politely and then directly and firmly stating your point or (counter)opinion. Kill them with kindness, and always remember to keep your manner and tone professional.

Here are some tips for dealing with specific types of detractors:

- **Snipers:** When ignoring them doesn't work, confront them. Ask the sniper a question to clarify a nasty remark or off-handed comment.
- **Talkers:** Stop speaking and look directly at the talkers. When you capture their attention, smile, nod, and then continue.
- **Deadheads:** Look directly at them so they're aware you've perceived their projected lack of investment or interest. Step toward them and ask them a question. Get them involved.
- **Know-it-alls:** Even if their comment makes you swell with annoyance, thank them for their input and continue. Avoid eye contact with them, make a concerted effort to include others, and, if necessary, say, "Let's hear from those who haven't yet spoken."

When transitioning from college life to the professional work world, it is important to leave behind colloquial speech and informal jargon. So your *dude, no problem, what's up?* and the like should be shed like a too-small pair of shoes and exchanged for more classic, grown-up language.

Be wary, though, of trying to pepper your speech with high-falutin words when simpler ones will suffice. Avoid mumbling, talking too softly or too loudly, or speaking in a way that identifies you with a particular group or social class.

When speaking to persuade, try a face-to-face approach first; telephone communication is a second-best option, but e-mail is the least persuasive and should be used only as a last resort.

EXERCISE 1

Prepare a speech, and then present it in front of your webcam. Time yourself, and critique your presentation. Repeat it until you are comfortable with and confident in your delivery.

EXERCISE 2

Check out Toastmasters International (www.toastmasters.org), and attend one of their meetings.

RESOURCES

Gallo, C. 2014. *Talk Like TED: The 9 Public-Speaking Secrets of the World's Top Minds.* New York: St. Martin's Press.

Toastmasters International. 2014. "Public Speaking Articles." Accessed November 11. www.toastmasters.org/MainMenu Categories/FreeResources/NeedHelpGivingaSpeech.aspx.

Master Persuasive Presentations

Knowing how to speak persuasively empowers you.
If you are able to say what you think succinctly, engagingly,
and in a way that people can understand, then you will be able to
land a good job, persuade colleagues, connect with clients, and
impress your boss. There is no better feeling in the world than
knowing that you can say what you think, even under pressure,
and that people will listen. Anyone can master this skill—
if you take the time to practice it.

—*Molly Bishop Shadel, professor,*
University of Virginia School of Law, Charlottesville

AMONG THE MOST pervasive fears Americans face is trepidation about public speaking, and executives are no exception. Some degree of anxiety about public speaking is natural, but when that fear becomes an obstacle to career success, it's a problem that must be addressed. Extreme physiological responses to public speaking—sweating, shaking, stomach upset, and the like—are usually mitigated with a few simple exercises and a determination to practice, practice, practice.

Such public speaking exercises have been around since the time of Aristotle and center on three basic tenets of persuasion or rhetoric: ethos, pathos, and logos. The first, *ethos*, is the ability to convince your audience that you have good character and credibility. The following are simple tools to boost your ethos:

- **Do your homework.** Use the Internet to research different aspects of your topic, and synthesize why it's critical, newsworthy, and important to discuss. Keep a balanced point of view. If conflicting evidence or differing opinions surround the topic, know what they are—and how to address them.

- **Practice beforehand.** Your presentation should not appear memorized or robotic, but it should have a sense of rhythm and flow that show you are prepared. Go to a quiet space, close the door, and practice out loud. Time yourself. Don't be a slave to your notes. Tell illustrative stories. As you practice, remember to pause as you speak—and always, always remember to be yourself. Feign comfort, even if you don't feel it.

- **Be respectful to everyone and their points of view.** Humorous asides that you meant to be funny may in fact offend. Stories that you meant to be illustrative may have political overtones. Take charge of your body language, your tone, and your speech, and learn to disagree without giving offense. If appropriate, move on by taking in audience input with a nod and without offering your personal opinions. If an audience member says something with which you disagree, be respectful—and don't feel the need to expound your view right then and there at the head of the room. If you're speaking on a topic that's sensitive or controversial, imagine in advance the types of comments or questions you'll field, and practice how to answer them. You'll be glad you did.

- **Pay attention to delivery.** Let your gaze rove across the audience so that you don't appear to be speaking to one section of the room or to certain people—try to establish eye contact with everyone. But don't maintain eye contact too long with individuals lest you lose your train of thought; instead, learn to focus slightly above their eyes.

Use open body language, your hands, and mobility to animate your words, even if it feels artificial. If you're at a podium and are expected to remain there, stand firm on both feet without rocking, leaning, or putting your hands in your pockets. Try not to touch your face or play with your hair. Avoid filler sounds and words such as *um*, *and*, *you know*, and *things like that*, and try to sound comfortable and natural without being stiff. Consider practicing in front of a webcam or video camera so that you can increase your awareness of the filler sounds you use and practice eliminating them.

- **Activate your language.** If appropriate, use stories to grab people's attention or to illustrate a point. Engage your listeners with some back-and-forth. Be someone to whom *you'd* like to listen.

Pathos is engaging the emotions of your audience. As you prepare your remarks, consider the following:

- Why should your audience care about what you are saying?
- Why do *you* care about what you're saying?
- What tone, stories, or messages will engage an emotional response?

It's important to find an appropriate theme for your presentation and tie it to something you know well. But make an effort to know your audience, too. One mistake that novice speakers make is not knowing their audience and improperly gearing the content to the listeners. If you are addressing a group of employees from the dietary division, consider the focus of their work and why they should care about your topic. A room full of dietitians and nutritionists might receive a different tone or message than, say, a board of directors.

Logos is the ability to excite the mind with reason. Here is where you take the time to make your central points succinctly and fluently. Excellent speakers start by saying what they will be offering in their talk, then they say those things, and then they say (again) what they said. Listeners, no matter who they are, tend to have short attention spans and won't take away difficult concepts or recall long sentences. Think about your messages as newspaper headlines. If your audience is overwhelmed by dense, lengthy, Faulknerian sentences, they will lose your message and become unfocused, and you'll have lost your chance to convey what you wanted. Identify and group your takeaway messages into three to five points. During delivery, tell your audience what your points are at the beginning, and repeat them at the end. Use plain English, please, without highfalutin words—you don't get extra credit for being abstruse, and you'll seem snobby.

Although PowerPoint is useful in presentations, take care not to overly rely on the program. If you're using PowerPoint, include as few slides as you can. Simplify your message and the look of your content, using a consistent background color, typeface, and font size. Whatever you do, don't simply read what is on your slides, and don't look at the slides while you're talking. Look at your audience. And remember to smile while you're addressing them.

Finally, whether you're speaking for an hour or five minutes, remember to end on time—even if you have more slides or more to say. Your allotted time is better used offering up a few memorable points than trying to convince your audience how much you know about a particular topic or rushing to squeeze the last few slides in at a pace that is difficult to take in.

EXERCISE 1

Write a five-minute speech on a topic related to a problem in your organization for which you have a strong solution. Sell your solution using stories, outlining the problem's history, sharing your perspective on it, and explaining the details of your solution. If possible, record yourself and keep watch of the time. Once you've delivered the speech, examine it for weak points, noting mannerisms, foibles, and filler words that should be avoided. Attempt to be someone you'd want to hear speak.

EXERCISE 2

Refocus the speech in Exercise 1 for a different audience. How will you change the content? The delivery? Record yourself delivering the speech, and assess your effectiveness.

RESOURCES

Sayler, R. N., and M. B. Shadel. 2011. *Tongue-Tied America: Reviving the Art of Verbal Persuasion.* New York: Aspen Publishers.

Shadel, M. B. 2012. *Finding Your Voice in Law School: Mastering Classroom Cold Calls, Job Interviews, and Other Verbal Challenges.* Durham, NC: Carolina Academic Press.

Conquer Negotiating

When I'm negotiating, I try to understand all the points from the other side, as well as the perspective that surrounds them— but I ask that they do the same for me. If I give a little on price, which is important to them, I make sure they understand my contract limitations. Really listening to the other party is truly the key to a successful negotiation; and when you do that, everyone really can end up with most of what they want.

—*Doug Wetmore, partner, Ivy Ventures,*
Richmond, Virginia

SKILLFUL NEGOTIATION CAN improve any organization's bottom line. It can result in fair and reasonable labor rates, optimal staffing patterns, and lower costs—not just equipment and construction costs but the service costs of physicians, consultants, and others as well. Good negotiations can also improve revenues when working out reimbursement contracts.

Being a good negotiator contributes to your personal bottom line, too. When you are offered a new job, for example, negotiating prowess comes in handy in discussions related to salary, scope of responsibility, and deadlines for deliverables. If you can negotiate, you don't just take what you're handed; you assert yourself—and your wants and needs—firmly, eloquently, and always politely.

There's a popular idea that good negotiators are tough and hard-boiled and that their take-no-prisoners attitude and fearsome tactics are what really seals the deal. But railroading others isn't a best practice in *any* regard. The best negotiators listen, explain, and prepare. They are firm but kind. They don't act like jerks. They consider all possible directions a discussion might take before it happens. And they're ready for it.

Negotiations have a before, a during, and an after. During the prenegotiation phase, you'll decide the following:

- **Who will handle the negotiation:** Will a team represent your organization, or will a single person do so? The former has certain advantages: It forces preparation, allows team members to draw on one another's expertise, enhances listening skills, and provides an opportunity to caucus through focused discussion. A team also enhances interdisciplinary coordination because it allows you to assign someone to record what's said and by whom during negotiation.

- **What you need to accomplish:** Start with high (but reasonable) expectations, and stick to them. Success in negotiation is often linked to an ability to maintain high expectations while lowering the expectations of those you're negotiating with. But remember that goals must be realistic and supported by evidence. Aim high, but don't be unwilling to budge—know what outcome you would be willing to walk away with.

- **How to analyze your opponents' position:** First, scrutinize in advance their terms and conditions to fully understand what they're after. Then take it further: What are their unstated needs? Also consider what strategies and techniques have worked in the past and whom they will assemble to be part of their team.

- **What your strategy will be:** Decide how low you are willing to go in the event you need to settle. Just as you made sure your original goals are supported by facts and logic, make sure the low end of your expectations is realistic.

- **What the tone will be:** The tone you take is tricky because you don't want to be a pushover, but you don't want to be nasty either. Assume a moderate stance, if you can. You're not there to win at all costs, particularly if you are dealing with employees whose loyalty, skill, and goodwill are critical (traits that can easily be marred in the process), but you're not there to be dictated to either. Find a middle ground that's firm but polite.

- **What additional items might be brought to bear:** Especially in cases of new hires and human resources negotiations, have a few things in your pocket that may seem negligible but can sweeten the deal if the other side is required to dramatically lower their expectations. For example, if the nurses' union is asking for a 10 percent raise and you know the budget won't allow more than 3 percent, consider other ways to fortify the deal. Free parking is one; more paid time off is another. Don't be afraid to be unconventional in your approach because it's not always the money that matters—the gesture, the listening, and the thought often count just as much.

If you wish to be taken seriously, your opponent must perceive that you've got bargaining power. Otherwise, you will lack an edge in the process. You might have it by position, reputation, knowledge, or deadlines—but you should stand tall in your authority as a negotiator. That said, no one individual or team should be authorized to fully commit the institution at the negotiation table. In your preparations, work with those who have ultimate authority—the CEO, the CFO, and others—to know the ranges of give and take you plan to offer. Don't surprise them. All parties should know that it's not official until the boss signs on the dotted line.

The formal negotiation begins with an initial agreement about the meeting's agenda and procedures. Each side makes a presentation, and then a discussion follows. During this process, you should do the following:

- **Really listen to, understand, and acknowledge the opponents' position.** Let them talk first. Ask frank questions about their goals so that you can glean the acceptable ranges for settlement and ascertain which areas are flexible and which are less so. After you listen carefully, repeat what you heard, and ask them to confirm that your understanding is correct.

- **Present your arguments clearly and concisely.** When it's your turn, don't go into impossible details that may create the impression that you're trying to obfuscate. Keep it clear, concise, and short. Make your best arguments at the beginning and end.

- **Identify areas where you and your opponent agree— and where you disagree.** Do so periodically during the discussion. Use a respectful tone.

- **Assess what you'll concede in exchange for your opponent's concessions in other areas.** Be willing to give on issues that are less important to you but could be important to your opponent.

- **Move.** Don't utter the same points over and over again without seeming to budge. Splitting the difference can sometimes work you out of the inertia.

- **Justify.** As you make offers, be sure your opponent understands your position and justification.

- **Keep your concessions on a short leash.** When you concede, don't stray more than a few degrees from the numbers you decided on during your preparation. If you are discussing a raise, don't offer 3 percent and then agree to 10 percent. Too big a leap implies ineptitude and amateurishness. Make sure your "gives" are within a decent range.

Once an agreement has been reached, document it. Prepare a memorandum of understanding (MOU), which will serve as the basis for the formal written contract. The MOU doesn't need to be anything fancy, but it should include the main agreed-upon points. Don't sweat the minutiae at this point—those can be dealt with later. Have both parties sign the document.

As you negotiate, buoy your own practice with the following time-tested negotiation skills—and take note of them when you see them in others.

- **Emphasize mutual interest.** Constantly remind your opponent that the objective is to achieve an agreement that is in the best possible interests of both parties.
- **Express statements as questions.** Rather than saying, "We should handle this. . ." or "Your estimate of costs appears to be unsupported," you might instead ask, "How do you think we should handle this?" or "How do you support your estimate of costs?"
- **Keep quiet.** For many of us, silence is uncomfortable. Fight the urge to fill the void—it often encourages the opponent to talk more and reveal more about his position.
- **Go second, and start small.** Getting your opponent to make the first concession is usually advantageous. If you are the first to concede something, make it on an issue of minor importance.
- **Tit for tat.** For each concession you make, get one from your opponent.
- **Make the other side seem unreasonable.** You could perhaps say, "We've made a number of concessions; now isn't it your turn?"
- **Don't be a deadline slave.** Extend it, if necessary.

- **Be funny and engaging.** Doing so takes some of the weight off the process, creates a feeling of cohesion and compatibility, and makes a solution seem all the more appealing—and more likely.
- **Rally your caucus.** Leave the room with your team to discuss a concession or settlement—or take a break to restore order if the communication has become heated and tense.
- **Formally close the negotiation.** When you have reached agreement, strike while the iron's hot—assert that it offers the best solution for both parties, and then move swiftly to prepare and sign the MOU.

Negotiating is something to practice and get comfortable with. Although formal tactics can give you some pointers and ideas, no single path exists through a negotiation process that can be maddening, frustrating, and lengthy—yet sometimes even satisfying. Just remember that negotiations about items both big and small can be mediated through two tactics: buying time and limiting your authority.

So when the surgeon stops you in the hallway and asks you for a new piece of equipment, be honest about the fact that you'll have to do some research. Say you'll discuss it with your boss and get back to him. *And then do it.*

EXERCISE 1

Complete a continuing education seminar on negotiating, such as the one offered by ACHE (www.ache.org/seminars/seminar .cfm?PC=NEGOT).

EXERCISE 2

Practice the techniques outlined in this lesson the next time you are negotiating an equipment purchase. Reflect on the experience.

What did you change about your approach? Did it change the outcome?

RESOURCE

Laubach, C. L. 2002. *Mastering the Negotiation Process: A Practical Guide for the Healthcare Executive.* Chicago: Health Administration Press.

Manage Conflict

Addressing a conflict in a constructive manner
can actually produce a better outcome than if there
had not been a conflict at all. President Clinton
referred to this openness of thought as "a third way."

—*Chris Carney, CEO, Diamond Healthcare,*
Richmond, Virginia

IT GOES WITHOUT saying that you will experience conflict
throughout your life and career—there is honestly no avoiding it.
In many respects, your job as a healthcare executive will be to serve
as resolver-in-chief. Many of the best leaders are exactly this, and
they are trusted for their resolving skills.

Contrary to popular belief, conflict can be a boon when those
engaged in it feel strongly about an issue or project. It results in
productive discussions, and progress is often made because people
truly want to do what's best for the organization and relax their
demands a bit to earn peace. But if left unresolved or half-resolved,
conflict can turn destructive. People take sides and assign motives.
Problems that had a modest-sized root become overgrown, tangled,
and twisted. And although even these big, many-layered conflicts
eventually get resolved, the long, drawn-out process can not only
fatigue your employees emotionally but also damage productivity
and—ultimately and most importantly—patient care.

Endless sources of conflict exist within an organization. But true leaders manage a way out of the morass and enable everyone involved to get a little something they want while not acquiescing entirely to any one person. Here's how to be that beloved, problem-solving manager who isn't conflict averse.

- **Set a professional tone for everyday behavior and conflict resolution.** Never yell. Never throw objects. Never be openly hostile, even if faced with hostility. Insist on professional behavior from yourself and others. Keep calm even in the throes of conflict.
- **Determine what's *really* at the root.** If you can glean the conflict's source, you can solve the problem. Are poor communicators involved, or are their unresolved issues from the past reemerging? Is there a struggle for power and a clash of egos, or are people just having a bad day? If you take a hard look at the whys, the how will likely reveal itself.
- **Empathize with each side.** Poor communication and lackluster listening are major sources of conflict in organizations across the board. Listen thoughtfully to all parties involved, and convey that you understand both sides of a conflict (even if you favor one side over another). In the early moments of a conflict, never assume a side. Don't interrupt when others are talking. Ask questions, and repeat what you've heard.
- **Establish the central facts.** Sometimes a conflict arises and neither party understands what has really happened. Get the facts. Attempt to get everyone to agree on them.
- **Don't take it personally.** It's completely normal to have disagreements—even robust ones—with colleagues, bosses, and employees. Don't take cheap shots at someone for voicing an opposing opinion—and don't let others do so either. The best solutions often come from healthy,

frank, and professional debate. Always be respectful of the opinions of others—even if what they say sounds ludicrous to you. Don't judge.

- **Start with heart.** When hurt feelings have erupted between parties, acknowledge those feelings but emphasize that everyone involved really wants what's best for the organization—and, ultimately, for patients. Acknowledge that you feel the powerful pull of emotions, too, but that you have intense respect for and confidence in those with whom you work—and you know that everyone present has the best, most honorable intentions.

- **Be willing to go first.** State your position, followed by a simple, meaningful solution. Even if it feels half baked, offering a possible pathway out of the argument may help generate new, better ideas for resolving the issue.

- **Take a break, then reconvene.** If the conversation isn't going anywhere and you feel you're just spinning your wheels, take a break. Have conversations one-on-one at another time. But make sure to reach resolution in person rather than over the phone or by e-mail because people are usually more mild mannered when talking face-to-face.

- **Learn to pick your battles.** Decide what is really worth your time and energy. You do not have to resolve every conflict—many conflicts will resolve themselves. Do not get involved in gossip or idle speculation. Your concern is anything that prevents the organization from achieving its goals.

- **Seek counsel when you cannot work out a resolution.** If you cannot resolve a conflict, bringing in a third party may help solve the problem. Often, a fresh set of eyes and ears can offer solutions that have not previously been considered. It will help if the counselor has the respect of everyone involved.

You will experience conflicts during your career. Do not try to avoid them. Ideally, solutions will be permanent and systematic. Work hard to make sure that conflict does not become personal. The way you resolve conflict will be an important key to your success as a healthcare executive. Ongoing conflict can sap an organization of its energy—energy that should be focused on carrying out its mission.

EXERCISE 1

Practice listening to what others are arguing about without interrupting anyone—not once. Think about what they are saying and why they are saying it. Have they mentioned a possible solution to the conflict?

EXERCISE 2

Read one book and one article on conflict management. Talk to experienced managers about how they resolve conflict.

RESOURCES

Fisher, R., W. L. Ury, and B. Patton. 2011. *Getting to Yes: Negotiating Agreement Without Giving In,* revised edition. New York: Penguin Books.

Mangold, K., and C. J. Hahn. 2014. *Confidence in Conflict for Everyday Life: Proven Strategies for Conflict Resolution and Communicating Under Pressure.* Milwaukee, WI: Truths Publishing.

Commit to Integrity and Ethical Behavior

Frequently, we think of ethics and integrity as though
they were something outside of us, almost imposed on us,
when in reality I believe it is living out the best of who we are.
It is recognizing who we are called to be, and living out that call.
When we are true to ourselves and live out of our core,
others see that truth in us and trust us. We create an environment
of trust where our words and behaviors are one. This environment
of trust draws others to the safety of being truthful
and honest, which magnifies in the environment of trust.

—*Sister Patricia Eck, CBS,
congregation leader, Congregation of Bon Secours,
Marriottsville, Maryland*

HEALTHCARE IS UNLIKE any other profession and is a special
domain for a host of reasons. Because its core operation depends
on ethical behavior and integrity without interruption or fail,
how employees conduct themselves is consistently of paramount
importance—as is how the organization governs itself when things
or people go awry.

All healthcare executives must familiarize themselves with the
Code of Ethics of the American College of Healthcare Executives
(www.ache.org/abt_ache/code.cfm), which most graduate students in healthcare administration have encountered during their

coursework. The *Code of Ethics* contains standards of behaviors to guide an executive's professional relationships, including those with colleagues, patients or others served, members of the executive's organization and other organizations, the external community, and society as a whole. It also outlines standards of ethical behavior to guide individuals' conduct, particularly when that conduct directly relates to the role and identity of the healthcare executive.

Of course, ethics and integrity were part of your life well before graduate school. Nurtured by your family, friends, and teachers, your own personal code of ethics guided you through early life, informing your education, first jobs, and relationships. You have had a sense of right and wrong from childhood. But for working adults, issues are rarely as black and white as they are when we're kids. In life in general, and in the world of healthcare in particular, there can be many shades of gray.

In your work, as in life, there will be times when your personal code of ethics feels violated by another's actions. If this happens repeatedly, and without resolution or reconciliation, you're prone to what nurse researchers Ann Hamric and Elizabeth Epstein call the "crescendo effect"—a cycle of moral distress that you feel powerless to change. This cycle leads to burnout, disengagement, and ultimately physical, emotional, or psychological health issues. Some people even leave their profession altogether because of it.

Over the course of decades of teaching healthcare leadership classes, we've asked students of all ages and from all manner of backgrounds what they believe the most important leadership traits to be. Without exception, integrity is among the first mentioned. But although everyone seems to agree that integrity is a critical character trait, there is little consensus about what constitutes it or the specific behaviors that manifest it. Merriam-Webster defines *integrity* as "the quality of being honest and fair" and "the state of being complete or whole," but integrity goes a lot deeper than that.

So what can you do to ensure integrity and a spotless ethical character? Have an inner compass, and follow it. Also keep the following advice in mind:

- **Be authentic.** If you take the time to connect with people in real ways, it will lead to trust.
- **Tell the truth.** Tell it as you honestly see it, and base it on reality. And say what you mean: Let your yes mean yes, and your no mean no.
- **Hear people out.** Listen and synthesize what people tell you. Listening intently, particularly when it really matters, is a key ingredient in authenticity.
- **Keep your promises.** Do what you say you will do. Do it on time and in the manner promised. And keep your work quality consistently high—don't offer half-baked responses or shoddy work.
- **Embrace and deal with the negatives.** Admit up front when you are at fault, and if you owe someone an apology, offer it without hesitation. Listen to those who have experienced fallout from your decision making. Then assume a "where do we go from here?" stance, if appropriate.
- **Commit to growth and transformation.** Be a visionary, big-picture type, but never lose sight of those whom you depend on to get you there. In other words: See the big picture but pay attention to details and people.
- **Keep it classy.** In conflicts, don't hit below the belt, even if you feel like it. Consistently take the high road. Always keep your professional cool.
- **Acknowledge and disclose conflicts of interest.** Never accept gifts from a customer or vendor that you shouldn't. If it feels even slightly wrong, it is. Don't do it.
- **Behave.** Don't do anything that you wouldn't want your mother (or your boss) to read about on the front page of the newspaper.
- **Sync up.** Be sure your personal values align with the values of your organization.

- **Know the boundaries of your personal code of ethics.** Know where you'll compromise and where you'll draw your line in the sand.
- **Don't cave in to peer pressure.** You know right from wrong. Don't feel pressured to give in to what you see others saying or doing if you think it's wrong.

EXERCISE 1

Write down what you consider to be your five most important personal values.

EXERCISE 2

Write a personal code of ethics—a description of behaviors that reflect your values.

RESOURCES

Cloud, H. 2006. *Integrity: The Courage to Meet the Demands of Reality.* New York: HarperCollins.

Epstein, E. G., and S. Delgado. 2010. "Understanding and Addressing Moral Distress." *Online Journal of Issues in Nursing* 15 (3): Manuscript 1. doi:10.3912/OJIN.Vol 15No03Man01.

Filerman, G. L., A. E. Mills, and P. M. Schyve. 2013. *Managerial Ethics in Healthcare: A New Perspective.* Chicago: Health Administration Press.

Perry, F. 2013. *The Tracks We Leave: Ethics and Management Dilemmas in Healthcare,* second edition. Chicago: Health Administration Press.

Look the Part

As an early careerist, it is important to represent yourself
as confident and detail oriented. The perfect way to set that
tone is with your dress. This is not to say you need to be
in an expensive suit each day, but the details do matter. Clean,
pressed clothing that matches and fits well signifies that you
take pride in yourself and how you portray your organization.

—*Greg Dadlez, MHA,*
clinical manager, Ochsner Clinic,
New Orleans, Louisiana

If you want to be a hospital CEO, dress like one—even if you're in
the first year of your career. Always remember that it's far better
to be overdressed than underdressed. And if you're questioning
whether your outfit is appropriate, it's likely not. Clothes aside,
keep in mind that a professional appearance is far more than
just your outfit. Confidence and a genuine smile go a long way.

—*Leigh T. Sewell,*
chief of staff and vice president, children's services,
Bon Secours Virginia Health System,
Richmond, Virginia

DURING COLLEGE OR graduate school, you might have been
able to let the haircut slide, not shave for a few days, wear the same
ripped jeans to class more than once, or go without shampooing

your hair during exam week by donning a hoodie. In the working world, of course, this is not a good idea. Good grooming and a professional appearance send a message that you are poised and confident and that you understand the unwritten rules of how to conduct yourself—and present yourself—in the workplace.

Usually, a student's first meaningful, full-time employment means the need to consider and invest in a professional appearance. Previously, one good business interview suit, a sport coat or two, or a handful of appropriate dresses and heels were sufficient. Now you need to wear business attire five days a week (with time built in to send and retrieve outfits from the dry cleaners). And although it doesn't matter exactly how many clothes you have, you should look the part each and every day. And mostly, that means looking like you care.

Many offices have experienced great change in just a generation insofar as attire is concerned. Women no longer always wear dresses, heels, hats, and gloves, and men don't always don ties and sport coats. Even the leaders of large, well-regarded, multimillion-dollar organizations may lack a top-to-bottom formality in dress. Yet, leaders always keep their outfits classic and simple. You can't go wrong with that.

But dressing well means more than having an expensive suit or Italian-made slingbacks. Just as your mother told you, a great deal of beauty comes from within. If you dress well, pay attention to your grooming, cultivate a warm smile, and come across as friendly, articulate, and caring, you will be good looking on many fronts. Looks are all in the smile and the eyes. Smiles that light up a room are magnetic and powerful. Eyes that twinkle show you are full of life—and good ideas.

Beyond clothes are the other items: your posture, your stride, your handshake—even how you laugh. When you walk into a room, stand erect with your head held high. Look around at others and smile. Your handshake should be firm and confident. This is not the time to slouch, slump, or look scruffy. It's not the time to jiggle your legs out of nervous habit, bite your nails, swagger, chew gum, or twirl your hair. Own the skin you're in, even if you feel like you're faking it. Confidence is 100 percent appealing, even if you feel only 35 percent self-assured.

Here are some additional pointers for maximizing your professional appearance:

- For both men and women
  - Take your dress cues from other, more senior administrators. Follow their degree of formality, considering regional and geographic variances in dress as well as rules for more casual wear (e.g., sandals, jeans on Friday). A job is not a fashion show—you're there to impress with your work—but you shouldn't make a bad impression by failing to adhere to unwritten dress code rules.
  - Clothes should be clean and pressed and fit well—nothing too tight, too short, too risqué, or with too many frills.
  - Wear cologne or perfume sparingly, if at all.
  - Make sure your hands are clean and your nails well manicured.
  - Keep your hair clean and well styled.
  - Keep a toothbrush at work, just in case you have pizza or onion soup for lunch; keep your teeth clean and your breath fresh as best you can.
  - Keep your shoes polished and non-scuffed.
  - Make sure leathers match (shoes and belt).
  - Cover tattoos and piercings (except earrings for women).
  - Keep jewelry to a minimum.

- For men
  - Dress as though it's a special occasion (which it is—every day). Convey through dress that you care and that you're confident and in control.
  - Shave every day, keeping facial hair (including ears and eyebrows) neatly trimmed.
  - Use collar stays on dress shirts to avoid the flyaway look.
  - Keep suits to conservative colors, such as navy blue, brown, or gray. Reserve black suits for big occasions, such as weddings and funerals. Choose stylish ties that hang low enough to touch the top of your belt buckle.
  - Shoes worn with suits should be lace-ups. Save the slip-ons and loafers for sport coats and dress pants. Socks should match the color of your suit pants.
  - Button-down collared shirts, khakis, and penny loafers are more collegiate than business professional. Avoid looking like a frat boy or college kid who just landed a job. It's time to look like a grown-up.
  - Pant cuffs should fall lightly over your shoes and should cover your socks when standing.
  - Shirt cuffs should extend a half inch beyond the sleeve of your suit jacket.

- For women
  - Necklines must always be conservative. No cleavage in the office—ever.
  - No suggestive fabrics, such as sheer blouses or lacy tops; you want to be taken seriously, and risqué dress is not worth the risk.
  - Skirt length should be conservative but stylish. Nothing higher than just above the knee. Classic pencil skirts look great on almost everybody.

- Bare legs are inappropriate, no matter what anyone tells you, in most office settings. Wear light stockings in summer, tights in winter.
- Keep makeup subtle and natural looking. Nothing too garish or heavily applied, especially in terms of eye shadow or lipstick.
- Sleeveless tops are fine in the height of summer as long as they're paired with a modest skirt or pants.
- Always wear a blouse—not a T-shirt, tank, or cami—with your suit.
- It's great to pair bold colors with more conservative ones (e.g., a brightly colored scarf with a dark suit). Bold accessories (e.g., big, chunky necklaces) are fine too, but if you wear something flashy, keep the rest of your outfit more muted.
- Keep the soles of your shoes fairly close to the ground, and try generally to wear closed-toe shoes. Extremely high heels and shoes with elaborate accessories are not proper office attire.
- Giant earrings, overly glitzy jewelry, or souped-up handbags are not appropriate either. Don't give anyone a chance to poke fun at your style (something that's more likely to happen to women than men). You don't want to be pigeonholed for your style—it will create more work for you in the long run, fairly or unfairly, for which you'll have to compensate.

Early in your career, you may not have the budget to completely revamp your wardrobe. But that doesn't mean you can't take a strategic approach and buy good-quality clothes that will be a smart long-term investment. For men or women, a well-made, nicely fitting navy suit (suit coat and pants or pencil skirt) is a great place to start. From there, you can begin to take over the world—and accessorize your way as you move up the career ladder.

EXERCISE 1

Take an inventory of your clothes and shoes. Have you worn them in the past year? Are they out of style? Develop a plan to purge clothes that no longer work for you, and budget for replacements. When suits start to look shiny, shirt cuffs fray, ties aren't crisp when tied, and socks have that worn area where the shoes rub, it is time to give them up.

EXERCISE 2

Identify someone you consider to be a snappy dresser, and ask them for advice about how to develop a wardrobe. They may also be able to refer you to a salesperson who can advise you on a wardrobe that fits your budget.

RESOURCES

Baumgartner, J. 2012. *You Are What You Wear: What Your Clothes Reveal About You.* Boston: Da Capo Lifelong Books.

Dye, C. F. 1993. *Protocols for Health Care Executive Behavior: A Factor for Success.* Chicago: Health Administration Press.

Gross, K. J., and J. Stone. 2002a. *Dress Smart Men: Wardrobes That Win in the New Workplace.* New York: Chic Simple.

———. 2002b. *Dress Smart Women: Wardrobes That Win in the New Workplace.* New York: Chic Simple.

Anticipate and Prepare

It is safe to say that nobody could have predicted the events that occurred during and after the shootings at Virginia Tech on April 16, 2007. Our organization had to respond without hesitation and under the most difficult of circumstances. Though we'd regularly practiced our disaster response plans, like most organizations we never thought we might actually have to use them. Our preparation, however, created a solid foundation that enabled us to anticipate needs and react with precision. The information we received and the needs of our patients changed by the minute during the response, and for many days after. These "in the moment" decisions were quickly analyzed and acted upon and, ultimately, ended up saving lives. While many difficult lessons were learned in the days and months that followed for our hospital, community, and nation, the basic lesson of the importance of being prepared and anticipating is one that never fails to resonate time and again.

The pace of work in most healthcare settings is fast and often unpredictable and can be a challenge for even the most seasoned executives. Your ability to properly prepare for and anticipate issues or problems will not only help you to make good use of valuable time, it will enable you to respond when situations change unexpectedly.

—M. Scott Hill, MEd, MHA, FACHE, president and CEO, Columbus Regional Health, Columbus, Georgia; and former CEO, Montgomery Regional Hospital, Blacksburg, Virginia

THE SCOUT MOTTO is "be prepared." Few things are as troubling as people who arrive to critical conversations like blank slates, needing to be brought up to speed, asking questions they should have considered long ago, and attempting late in the game to bring their understanding up to par. Even if unintentional, such behavior is not only rude but also taps morale and the bottom line. It withers confidence and goodwill. And it makes the time waster an object of frustration and, worse, of ridicule.

Not being a time waster means you're prepared for each and every conversation, meeting, task, and project. You've considered in advance what the issues are and how you'll face them. Even in the early days of determining a solution, you've got a few ideas in your head to share and offer direction, and you're well aware of what the challenges are. In short, you've cared enough to think through issues in advance so that you're fresh and ready to offer pathways toward a solution.

If you prepare for a test, a good grade usually follows. But if you wing it or hack and fake your way through, the result is usually panic and a failing mark. In healthcare, as elsewhere, it's critical that you learn to prepare and anticipate. Don't be a time waster— *be prepared.* It's really that simple.

For meetings, remember to do the following:

- **Arrive early and be ready to focus on the issue at hand.** Turn off your electronics, and give your colleagues your undivided attention.

- **Prepare.** Imagine ahead of time the questions you'll be asked that are in your domain. Know and anticipate problems you might encounter along the way that touch your area of responsibility.

- **Huddle with your team.** Convene with close staff prior to a big meeting to collaborate about what's being discussed and to imagine together the different questions, routes, and solutions you plan to present. Several heads are often better than one.

- **Follow up.** If you're asked a question you can't answer, find the answer—and promptly report back.

Each day, try to do the following:

- **Plan longer-term.** Prepare for the next day's activities at the end of each day, and anticipate the next five days by outlining in your mind or on paper what generally will need to be touched, accomplished, and considered. If you're working on longer-range projects—for example, establishing an initiative that's to be launched six months or a year down the road—map out in advance how you'll get there and what tasks will need to be addressed along the way. Put electronic reminders to yourself in your calendar to prompt progress toward your goal.
- **Feel people out.** Take time to understand what your team thinks about the issues and projects before them, and know the decision maker's perspective, too. Early discussions will help you understand possible solutions and sense when there's a consensus. The most successful leaders have a good idea of how a discussion or vote will go prior to any discussion. If a key individual has strong feelings or a big stake in an issue, consider their view before raising the topic at a meeting.
- **Be of service.** Know what your boss is working on, and consider ways you can help, no matter how small. Making copies? Getting water? Taking coats? Small things can really make a difference.
- **Don't surprise anyone.** If you have bad news to share, be sure to inform all stakeholders. Tell your boss. Discuss the parameters of how to inform others in a calm,

solution-oriented way. While not minimizing bad news, keep your comments factual and then move quickly to solutions.

- **Prepare for the unexpected—and don't be derailed by it.** It's a truism that in life you can't prepare for everything. Having a good understanding of the culture and goals of your organization will help you when the unexpected happens. If you've overlooked something or made an error, own it and say how you'll remedy it—for example, "I didn't speak with Dr. Nice about the project, but I will reach out to get her input when I return to my desk."
- **Review how well you prepared at the end of each day.** Learn from mistakes and do better tomorrow.

If you're able to cultivate a reputation as someone who prepares for and anticipates problems and their solutions, you'll have a leg up on many in your organization who will consider you a go-to. Flying by the seat of your pants through any task or issue is never advisable, and preparation and anticipation will help make you a remarkable and effective executive.

EXERCISE 1

Develop a list of what you wish to accomplish at the beginning of each day, making sure you're prepared to tackle each item. For longer-term projects and goals, plot what you'll need to do each month to get there efficiently and on time.

EXERCISE 2

Make a list of priorities for yourself, your boss, and your organization over the next year. What small tasks can you omit from your daily routine that will allow you to focus on more important priorities?

RESOURCES

Babauta, L. 2009. *Zen Habits: Handbook for Life.* CreateSpace Independent Publishing Platform.

Cartwright, T., and Center for Creative Leadership. 2007. *Setting Priorities: Personal Values, Organizational Results.* San Francisco: Pfeiffer.

Build Resilience

Knowing you can overcome it means you will.
Smiling while you do it makes it easier. Believe—and enjoy.

—Carolyn C. Carpenter, MHA, FACHE,
associate vice president, Duke University Health System,
associate dean and administrator, Duke Cancer Institute,
Durham, North Carolina

WE ALL LEAD busy personal and professional lives, with stress swirling all around us. Nowadays, a certain amount of chaos, intense activity, and drama must be taken for granted. But it's *how* we handle and defuse stress—and what inner resources we tap in the process—that reveals our true mettle and is a real key to success.

It's fascinating to observe how some who have faced almost incredible hardships and tragedy are able to move beyond them, turning negatives into opportunities for growth and change. On the flip side, others never seem to fully recover from traumas such as divorce, the death of a loved one, or being fired. What accounts for the difference? How do some people harness resilience and perspective whereas others cannot?

A story to illustrate: A nursing student encountered one of his first patients, a man named Bill, who had been diagnosed with sarcoidosis, a chronic, incurable disease. Bill had lived with the disease for a long time and periodically spent time in hospitals for what he termed "tune-ups." When answering questions about his illness and how his life had changed, Bill was resolute and open: He found strength in faith and prayer and remembered to be grateful for each day, for being able to spend time with his large family, and for the opportunities his remaining days would bring. These were not just the canned utterances of a man who had heard or read such sentiments before; they were qualities evident in his engagement in the present, in his ability to accept and move beyond his tragedy with an uncanny level of beauty and grace. Few would deny that Bill had mastered the ability to face his illness head-on, find meaning in it, and do the best he could with the time he had to live. After he died, Bill's message of resilience never left the student.

Resilience really is about choosing the path of hardiness rather than the one of festering stress. Those who live with high levels of stress and unhappiness often give away their power to reframe the situation and harness control over it. They wait for others to change, or they focus on a situation or an event that they cannot control to the near exclusion of everything else. They're dissatisfied, disappointed, and disillusioned, and their bodies, minds, and families suffer as a result. They're more victims than victors.

These people come with a cost. When others attempt to reframe what's upsetting them and offer suggestions to ease the stress, these individuals resist. Their negativity bleeds out, sucking away the energy and momentum of others—even of whole organizations. They've missed the message that *at any point in life* resilience can actually be learned and followed.

Organizations can be resilient (or not) as well. Companies that are able to face reality, to turn negatives into opportunities, and to nimbly regroup and resource a turnaround will always have the competitive edge. In contrast, organizations that deny problems, shy away from risk, and never make plans to deal with future potential hardships will ultimately suffer and die. In today's dynamic, fast-changing healthcare environment, it's critical to be the former.

Being resilient begins with harnessing a positive attitude and practice, being willing to thoughtfully change, and being ready to move and find solutions without getting stuck in the quicksand of inertia. Some healthcare organizations even practice resilience engineering, a new approach to patient quality and safety that involves sustaining required operations under expected and unexpected conditions. Such exercises truly show an organization's—and a team's—ability to think on its feet through a crisis. Such activities might even turn stressed-out organizations into resilient ones.

So how to bring resilience to your personal life and infuse it in your organization?

- **Face reality.** This goes beyond mere optimism. In dire situations, rose-colored glasses may make the situation worse. Adopt a down-to-earth view of a problem's components, identify and own your and others' role in them, and determine realistically what basic steps are required for survival. This process can be practiced as an exercise—as with resilience engineering—or deployed when facing a real problem in real time.

- **Seek meaning from adversity.** Rather than asking, "Why is this happening?" ask, "What will I learn by suffering through this?" You may find the meaning of true friendship and discover strengths you never knew you had as you wade through adversity. The experience will inform the way you solve problems in the future.

- **Keep your values close.** Keeping your ideals close infuses your environment with purpose and meaning, enabling you to shape and interpret events. Keeping focused on an organization's values is even more important for organizational resilience than resilient employees are. Knowing what you (or your organization) will do—and what you (or it) won't do—to solve the problem will inform the best route out of it.

- **Be resourceful.** *Pluck* is when you make do with what you have on hand—and being resilient in this regard (rather than bemoaning what your deficits are) is important. Being nimble and able to improvise keeps you on the up-and-up, focused on solutions, and moving forward.

- **Rewrite negative scripts.** Or, as a friend might say, "If you don't like the play you're in, change the set." How you take responsibility as you respond to change puts the onus of control squarely on your shoulders. Don't wait for others to change or merely hope that events will unfold in your favor. Be thoughtful and active in making it better.

- **Accept yourself—and others.** Come to terms with your tendencies, strengths, and vulnerabilities, and forgive yourself and others for their foibles. Lead an authentic life that is consistent with your values. Stand tall in who you are—and be the best version of that person you can.

- **Own your mistakes—and then move on.** Rather than blame everything else when things go awry, admit your mistakes and your role in them, and then figure out how to proceed. An error is not confirmation that you are a failure—and it doesn't mean you're unfit for decision making. Sit up straight, apologize (if necessary), and then move on.

- **Be resilient in your life.** Your mother was right. Get enough sleep, eat right, exercise, and be kind to yourself, particularly as you cope with potential stressors.

Although tapping inner resilience may feel more awkward to some than to others, *every* person and *every* organization can learn it—with practice and the determination and understanding at the outset that change is required.

EXERCISE 1

Write a few paragraphs about a "negative script" in your life. How might you define a new role for yourself? What steps should you take to implement that role? What obstacles might interfere? What is your backup plan?

EXERCISE 2

List three situations where you made a mistake or failed at something. Recall how you explained these failures to others and to yourself. What was the worst thing that happened after you made the mistake? In the future, how might you reframe your mistakes and failures?

RESOURCES

Brooks, R., and S. Goldstein. 2004. *The Power of Resilience.* Chicago: Contemporary Books.

Coutu, D. L. 2002. "How Resilience Works." *Harvard Business Review* 80 (5): 46–55.

Hollnagel, E., J. Braithwaite, and R. L. Wears. 2013. *Resilient Health Care.* Burlington, VT: Ashgate Publishing Company.

Manage Your Job

I (KEN) HAVE had *two* best jobs. At the very beginning of my career, starting when I was 18 and for the next five years, I worked as an emergency room orthopedic technician in a Tulsa, Oklahoma, hospital. Responding quickly as part of a team that worked incredibly well together to allay our patients' fears and make them comfortable satisfied my itch to give the very best of myself to our patients. We team members (still in touch to this day) were not only proud of our roles; we also all felt we were part of something bigger than ourselves. To an 18-year-old college kid aching to find his way, the job offered an incredible vantage and beginning.

My current position at the University of Virginia (UVA) School of Nursing—I'm associate dean for strategic partnerships and innovation and hold the UVA Medical Center endowed chair in nursing—has been similarly gratifying because I get to spend my days doing what I love most and do best. This job offers autonomy and independence as well as teamwork and camaraderie, and my boss is a visionary and champion without being a micromanager. That I am valued as a person first and foremost, rather than as a producer or a product, is affirming—and brings out, I believe, my and my colleagues' best performance.

Steve's best job of all time was as CEO of Henrico Doctors' Hospital, a position he held for 16 years and one in which he felt a clear sense of alignment between authority and responsibility during a time of massive growth and change. The medical and hospital staff focused on improving patient care at every moment, and great teamwork was the order of the day.

But it was a much earlier job, when Steve was just 23, that really informed his ideas about servant leadership and influenced every position held later in his life. As a platoon leader during the Vietnam War—a time of incredible, poignant change and growth for our nation—Steve led young men in and out of combat, nurturing them in life and in survival. It forever changed him—in a *good* way.

Of course, like everyone, we've also both worked in terrible jobs—under lackluster, narcissistic, ineffective, and temperamental bosses; surrounded by bad conditions; and among unmotivated peers. We've both received superficial performance reviews, had bosses and colleagues who didn't listen, experienced ego-driven personalities, and seen some of the messiest offices in existence. We've both stayed too long in positions, hoping for a turnaround or some luck; and at other moments, we've left too soon for what we thought was a better opportunity that ultimately was not.

All of it, the good and the bad, influenced our paths, this book, and especially this section, Manage Your Job. You're knee-deep in developing your *own* track record, your *own* battery of references, and your *own* professional experiences and burgeoning skills. You can take charge of your career—but only if you manage yourself first, and your job second.

So now that you've landed the job you were looking for, how will you make it yours?

—Ken White

Own the Job You're In

Consider every experience, position held, and interaction
to be an opportunity to learn and grow. Focus on the task,
discussion, role, and job at hand with the intent to do them
all well. It is important to be intentional and purposeful in
your actions because everything you do has meaning. Begin
to know yourself, and seek opportunities based on who you
are, not always focusing on who you want to be. One would be
amazed how my roles as a secretary, a paralegal, and a nurse
have helped me be of service in various leadership roles within
the healthcare field. Realize the next step will always come!

*—Michelle Hereford, MSHA, RN, FACHE,
chief, community hospitals and post-acute care division,
University of Virginia Health System, Charlottesville*

MANY EARLY CAREERISTS spend inordinate time and energy
thinking about and jockeying to get a better, more advanced job
before mastering the position they're in. But *every* job has something valuable to teach, whether it's one you plan to keep for two
years or two decades. So the best way to advance your career is to
do a great job in the position you're in. You don't want to leave a
job before you've given it your all and absorbed the lessons it has to
impart. Remember to focus on what's right in front of you before
sprinting off in another direction that may (or may not) offer more
promise.

So how do you dig into the job you have?

- **Take your organization's mission and vision and "microtize" them to your area of responsibility.** You're there to add value. So it's important to understand your role in helping the organization achieve its objectives. Step one is to fully understand your company's current priorities as well as its overall strategy and direction. If it's focused on quality improvements, consider what you can do to help reduce errors or increase patient satisfaction. If its aim is to expand programs to deal with population health problems, mull over how you might help initiate and lead such growth.

- **Endeavor to go beyond what's expected.** After you're clear on your organization's goals and expectations—being sure to ask for clarification if needed—visualize how a successful year in your position might look. Figure out what you will need to move beyond what's expected of you, and leverage opportunities to exceed expectations. For example, if you recruit a new surgeon doing a novel, much-needed procedure, the increased revenue from the surgeon's activities may help you exceed your profit goals. If you can find two or three such levers, you may be able to plow through and exceed your goals. When your boss asks you for something, get it in on time and give more than was requested. Anticipate what the next logical step will be, and get on it.

- **Change something visible early on.** When you take a new job, try to accomplish something visible in your first few weeks. Rearrange the furniture, paint the reception room, start daily tours, or initiate a morning team coffee-time huddle. Talk to your supervisor to find out what's important. Based on what you learn, write out a 30- to 90-day action plan to make an impact, and share your plan with colleagues and supervisors. Keep everyone informed of the progress you make in implementing the plan, and be an expert at managing the details.

- **Be detail oriented.** This point can't be overstated. You want to make a great first impression—and honestly, you get one shot—and nothing ruins your chances of making that impression more than sloppily done, ill-conceived, error-ridden work. Make sure that what you produce is professional in appearance and that it's in the format your supervisor wants. Double-check your facts, spelling, and grammar. And complete your work on time. If you need more time, be transparent about it and discuss an extension. Be certain that your work solves problems and doesn't produce additional tasks for someone else or lead to more questions that need answering. Remember, too, that when your supervisor requests a report on a subject, she is asking you to define what this subject means to your organization. Be prepared to give thoughtful, well-researched, in-depth answers, not broad ones.

- **Keep your nose clean.** Don't waste time on gossip or office politics. Idle speculation can do harm. Off-the-cuff remarks and jokes are inappropriate, and work isn't the place for them. If others engage in them, don't get sucked in. Keep focused on your job. Surround yourself with others who do the same. And don't use profanity, even if you think it. It's never appropriate in a healthcare setting, and certainly not from an executive.

- **Ferret out strong colleagues.** Early on in a job, it usually becomes clear who your go-to resources are. Figure out who can help you succeed.

- **Plan ahead.** Anticipate what the organization and your supervisor will need. Think ahead and solve problems.

The best executives focus on the job in front of them. They give their best effort, thoughtfully solve problems, and invest the time and energy it takes to really tackle a job. And when they do that, promotions and opportunities invariably follow.

EXERCISE 1

Review the American College of Healthcare Executives (ACHE) Healthcare Executive Competencies Assessment Tool, and identify areas of strength and weakness. Develop an action plan to turn three weaknesses into strengths.

EXERCISE 2

Ask yourself, "How am I adding value to my job and organization?" How will you be remembered after you have left the organization? Write down ways you would like to be remembered, and then work and behave in ways to make it happen.

RESOURCES

American College of Healthcare Executives (ACHE). 2013. *ACHE Healthcare Executive Competencies Assessment Tool 2014.* www.ache.org/pdf/nonsecure/careers/competencies _booklet.pdf.

Drucker, P. F. 2004. "What Makes an Effective Executive?" *Harvard Business Review* 82 (6): 58–63, 136.

Dye, C. F., and A. N. Garman. 2015. *Exceptional Leadership: 16 Critical Competencies for Healthcare Executives,* second edition. Chicago: Health Administration Press.

Maximize the First 90 Days

The first three months of anyone's career are a critical period of adaptation and acceptance, absorption, and understanding. It's an important time to glean who the most important players are—those whose jobs directly touch yours and key stakeholders' in particular—and the point at which you'll determine how to best interact and communicate with them. But it's also a period during which to connect with *everyone* around you. Some combination of thoughtful listening and silence, observation, and action are critical during the first 90 days of any job. Only after that period of induction is action required.

—*Alan Keesee, FACHE,*
chief operating officer, Capital Regional Medical Center,
Tallahassee, Florida

IN THE US NAVY, when a new captain takes over a ship, the entire crew assembles to see a physical manifestation of the change of command. The new captain boards the ship as the retiring one disembarks, usually after a handshake and wave, in a ceremony that takes place under the gaze of all the sailors. It is abundantly clear who is now in charge.

Although you may not have the luxury of such a definitive induction ceremony in your new job, a proper beginning will ensure a successful tenure. A rocky start can mean a poor fit or be difficult to recover from—but not always. As the old saying goes, you have but one chance to make a good first impression, so it's important to start a new job carefully, thoughtfully, and properly.

Here are a few ideas to guide you in those early days:

- **Understand your role.** Before your first day, you should have a good idea of what those who hired you expect of you. What are the parameters of your authority and responsibility? Whom do you supervise? What's detailed in your official job description, and which responsibilities of yours may not be so clearly delineated? With time, of course, your role will become more sharply defined—but in those early days, if you are not sure what is expected, ask. Be frank about things that seem confusing or vague. As you gather information, goals—for yourself and for your organization—will likely crystallize.

- **Articulate your expectations to your staff—and the organization at large.** Call a department meeting early on, and ask for introductions and short background summaries from your colleagues. Offer some information about yourself as well before outlining your general concept of management. Listen attentively, and, above all, be friendly and do your best to appear comfortable even if you don't entirely feel it. Early impressions are often lasting impressions—and it's the rare person who's an affable combination of leader and mentor, listener, and strategist. Do your best to be that person.

- **Observe, listen, and ask.** You'll likely be leading some who are older than you and who have years of rich professional experience and perspective. These employees are often the people from whom you can glean the best, most pertinent, and most useful information. Such people are potent allies, too, and some may have seen many executives come and go. Get them on your side by being a thoughtful, responsive listener. Ask them about their projects, and see if they have ideas for improving things. Often, people have been waiting for someone to ask their opinion—and they'll relish the chance to offer it. Really listen to the responses you get. The most proficient executives learn to observe, listen, and ask questions well before they act.

- **Study the history and culture of your organization.** Savvy executives will alter their focus and approach based on current environmental realities. Tap a few colleagues as advisers who can help you during your first few months to fully understand the organization, where its roots lie, and where it's headed.

- **Gather information for at least a couple of months before instituting change.** Try to find out if the organization has any pressing problems that must be immediately addressed. If so, you may not have the luxury of delaying decisions. Otherwise, wait to act while you gather information.

- **Set goals for yourself and the organization as you begin your new position.** Try to determine what actions are necessary to ensure the organization's success. Here are a few critical questions to guide your goals: What are the most important existing and potential revenue sources? Who are your best and most important customers? Don't try to set too many goals at once—between three and five at the outset are probably enough. As you're marking them, be sure to clearly communicate the goals to the organization, your boss, and your colleagues.

- **Show leadership and professionalism in everything you do.** Your employees and colleagues will be watching and evaluating everything you do, say, and write. Be deliberate, but be careful and wise, too. Remember your manners, don't interrupt, and be unfailingly polite. And do your best to remember people's names.

- **Communicate! Communicate! Communicate!** Start your tenure by being a clear and honest communicator. People should understand your messages and will appreciate your transparency. And talk the talk. Be certain that when you say yes, you follow through. The same goes for saying no. If you can't do anything about a problem, say so. Your candor will be remembered—and appreciated.

- **Be visible.** All employees like to see their leaders. On the first day or two, visit all areas of the organization, from the common areas to the labs. Visit areas that do not often get attention, such as the boiler room, the surgical suite, the cafeteria or kitchen, and the loading dock. Word that there is a new leader traipsing around will quickly spread. And while you're being visible, introduce yourself to everyone you meet. Ask them what they do for the company, what they like about it, and what they dislike. You should continue these rounds—a critical part of what the best leaders do—throughout your tenure.

- **Ask routinely for a status report from *all* of your stakeholders.** Asking only your high-level advisory group how things are going might not reveal the entire picture. Ask a variety of people, "How are we doing? What mistakes are being made? What can we do better?"

Good planning and execution will ensure that you start your new position in good order. And a good start often leads to a good tenure.

EXERCISE 1

Keep a journal of events that happen in the first 90 days of your tenure, and set a goal for personal action during that period. When you have finished the first 90 days, set your sights on goals for the next 90 days.

EXERCISE 2

During the first 90 days, make a list of all the people you would like to meet during "listening rounds." When you meet with each one, jot down key discussion points. Ask, "What three things work really well here?" and "What three things don't work so well?" Before ending each meeting, ask, "Is there anyone else you think I should meet with or get to know?"

RESOURCES

Stein, M., and L. Christiansen. 2010. *Successful Onboarding: Strategies to Unlock Hidden Value Within Your Organization.* New York: McGraw-Hill.

Watkins, M. 2013. *The First 90 Days: Proven Strategies for Getting Up to Speed, Faster and Smarter.* Boston: Harvard Business Review Press.

Leverage Differences

Diversity initiatives often fall short of creating real change
because they overemphasize controlling or "managing"
diversity rather than exploiting or "leveraging" differences.
In any diverse environment, leaders succeed when they
capitalize on important differences rather than ignore them.

—*Martin N. Davidson, PhD,*
professor of leadership, Darden School of Business,
University of Virginia, Charlottesville,
and author of The End of Diversity as We Know It

AMERICA IS INCREASINGLY a melting pot of richly varied cultures, backgrounds, ethnicities, and points of view. As healthcare leaders, our purpose is to improve health and provide quality care to these diverse communities while recognizing, as we hire and promote, that our employees should reflect those they serve. Naturally, patients and their families feel most comfortable when those caring for them speak the same language and share a similar heritage or even common physical features. Medical centers and clinics would be prudent to make a concerted effort to connect with a wide variety of patients through thoughtful planning, recruitment, and hiring practices.

In that spirit, the notion of diversity for diversity's sake is no longer the goal—diversity is simply good business. With a diverse patient base, hospitals can grow their market share by expanding and highlighting their cultural sensitivity and accommodation as well as the diversity of their workforce—management included. Healthcare organizations have pivoted away from defensiveness and become aggressively opportunistic as many place a growing focus on diversity. And although older executives are often used to certain types of people occupying certain roles, younger executives have become comfortable with diversity because they've grown up with it. In many ways, we're on the right path.

Historically, diversity referred to physical traits that were visible—gender, ethnicity, race, and age, for example. Diversity's modern definition, however, is more than skin deep. Notable among those calling for change in the way diversity is considered is business professor Martin Davidson, who argues that by considering people's diversity of perspective, experience, and strategy—rather than just their skin color or religion—an organization can widen and strengthen its talent pool. Davidson joins a growing chorus of individuals hoping to tap differences that aren't so obvious, including generational and religious differences as well as those relating to physical ability, sexual orientation, and even geographic origin, among others. It's time, asserts Davidson, for a sea change in the way we leverage diversity: Rather than merely aiming to buoy our numbers of women or racial minorities, we should consider diversity as a way to gain a breadth of perspectives different from our own and to break from tradition.

If you surround yourself with people exactly like you, harmony might ensue (boredom, too), but your growth and potential for innovation will stagnate. In contrast, if you pepper your team with people who bring different ways of thinking—based on their economic background, their political or religious views, or their sexual orientation, for example—you'll look through a wider, sharper, more nuanced lens. The work might be messier, but the outcome of a diverse team is often true innovation born of the ability to develop strategies from differences. The best, most effective teams aren't filled with yes-men; they're filled with those open to others' wisdom and perspective, who have the ability to consider all avenues before collaborating toward a solution. The result is often innovative and different—and highly successful.

Only when we harness and take into account our differences can we create better, more thoughtful healthcare systems and services for our patients—as well as develop and sustain an organizational culture that identifies strength in differences and promotes inclusion in the workforce. So where do you begin?

Start with yourself. Are you inclusive in your language? Are you mindful of and sensitive to others around you? After this self-reflection, consider the following ideas, which may help you be more mindful of ways to appreciate differences in and among people:

- **Generational:** Although certain generations tend to share some values and attitudes, never assume that certain characteristics "go" with a particular age group. For example, don't assume that your older employee won't be technologically savvy or that your Gen X colleague is a depressed, latchkey child of divorce. Be cognizant of how different generations perceive change, technology, communication, and work–life integration—but be sure to acknowledge the individual, not the tenets of the generation to which he belongs (see Lesson 28 for more on generational differences).

- **Gender:** Men and women face different challenges in the workplace, and they often work differently and distinctly from one another. Many women (and some men) work full-time while raising a family. If you've got a talented employee, let her go on and off the fast track to leadership development while she's raising children, especially in the early years. Talent is rare and worth keeping, and by offering flexibility to working parents early on, you'll not only earn their loyalty over time—you'll also find these individuals are often wizards at time management. Once their children are older and more self-sufficient, these moms and dads will likely be among your best assets—and they'll bring an important perspective as parents to boot.

- **Caregivers:** Similar to caregivers of young children but dramatically less heralded, some workers have the responsibility of caring for their aging or infirm parents. These individuals have both special needs and perspectives that can be hugely important for a healthcare setting. Tap them for their wisdom, and continue to ask how they're doing and how their parent is faring. Building loyalty will boost caregivers' confidence that their perspective is critical—that they're valued not only for their work but also for their special vantage on the aging process and its inherent challenges.

- **Minorities and other cultures:** Aim to offer extra support to new minority hires and to employees from different cultures, and be interested and inquisitive (without being obtrusive) about their perspectives, traditions, and back stories. Have initiatives that support talented minority employees—such as formal mentorship programs or flexibility to attend religious or ethnic functions that may not be on everyone's calendar—to be sure you keep them.

- **Disabilities:** One of the nation's largest minority groups consists of people with disabilities. Providing special physical or emotional support to employees living with disabilities and to those caring for family members with disabilities enhances organizational sensitivity. Such support might be something as simple as walking alongside a slower-moving colleague with multiple sclerosis during a fire drill, allowing the parent of a child with cerebral palsy to telecommute, or holding the door for a peer who uses a cane. If you just think about the ways, large and small, that you can make life easier and more pleasant for those dealing with disabilities, you'll cultivate warmth and loyalty—and your organization will be the better for it.

- **LGBT** (lesbian, gay, bisexual, and transgender): Whether LGBT professionals self-identify or not, they're often overlooked in traditional diversity programs. To promote an inclusive and accepting work environment, sponsoring Safe Space training programs may be useful. Be an example of acceptance and warmth when you meet same-sex partners and spouses—others will take their cue from your behavior and follow suit.

- **Veterans:** Most veterans have great skills but experience difficulty in getting a chance to apply them in the workplace. Roughly 1 percent of the American population has served in the armed forces, and many individuals and organizations already make a concerted effort to support veterans in other ways. Offering them work may be one of the best ways to salute them.

As you aim to support those working in your organization who are different from you, remember that *what* you say and *how* you say it are often just as important as your actions. Use inclusive language, be sensitive to differences, and be careful not to offend. If you don't know the best way to demonstrate inclusion through language, ask.

Using nonspecific words such as *significant other*, *partner*, or *spouse* is the best way to invite couples to the summer barbeque or staff retreat luncheon. Avoid slang and derogatory words entirely. Being openly supportive of your rich variety of colleagues will prompt others around you to do the same.

And know your people. Even if your organization is a big one, make an effort to know a little about everyone on a personal level. Be accepting about who they are, where they come from, and what they bring. Doing so will push your organization's ethos in the direction of acceptance and transform it into a place that's successfully leveraging the differences within.

EXERCISE 1

Study whether the makeup of your staff reflects that of your clientele or patient base.

EXERCISE 2

Learn more about people who are different from you. Spend time getting to know them. Read about and learn ways you can be more sensitive to others in the words you use.

RESOURCE

Davidson, M. N. 2011. *The End of Diversity as We Know It: Why Diversity Efforts Fail and How Leveraging Difference Can Succeed.* San Francisco: Berrett-Koehler Publishers.

Organize Your Workspace

With a continuing increase in the volume and speed
of e-technology, it's easier to lose control of incoming
communications and priorities—and thus fail to meet
the expectations of clients, coworkers, and superiors—
so a well-organized environment is more critical than
ever. Being tidy for the sake of tidiness is not the point;
the point is enhancing opportunities for success in an
increasingly demanding healthcare environment.

—*Lawrence Prybil, PhD, LFACHE,
Norton Professor in Healthcare Leadership
and associate dean, College of Public Health,
University of Kentucky, Lexington*

YOU MAY BE an exceptional time manager and a beloved boss,
and you may set robust priorities—but what's in the top drawer of
your desk? How does your desktop (both literal and technological)
appear at the beginning, middle, and end of the day? How organized is your briefcase, handbag, or glove box, and how filthy is
your office coffee mug?

Although successful and professionally gifted individuals
occupy the entire spectrum of tidiness and organization—from
neat-freak immaculates to scattered and downright slobs—how
well you keep house in your office says a lot about you. Improving your organization level may have a positive impact on your

productivity, efficiency, stress level, and overall effectiveness. All it takes is being thoughtful, regimented, and neat!

The first question to ask is how you feel your office space is working for you. Can you find what you need when you need it? Do you have systems in place that help you prioritize, recall important meetings and events, and tally what you've done versus what still needs doing? Do you have files for bigger-picture projects and logs for inspiring articles and ideas that might inform your organization's wider vision and goals? And if you don't, do you mind?

If you're like many of us, your office could use some real thought and tidying up. Here are a few questions to consider at the outset:

- Are your desk, computer monitor, chair, and ancillary furniture (guest chairs, lighting, shelves, and so on) configured appropriately?
- Is your phone situated relative to your handedness (i.e., to the right if you're right-handed)?
- Are your trash can and recycling bin both accessible to you and cloaked from others?
- Is your furniture comfortable and ergonomically designed so that your posture is preserved?
- If it's useful in your role, do you have a place to meet other than your desk and a guest chair (a small table with chairs, perhaps)?

Your office says a lot about you—including its physical appearance, setup, and organization—so try to imagine the picture it conveys, and decide whether that picture matches the one you want people to take away as an impression when they meet with you there.

Your office should also serve as a haven for you to do good work with minimal distractions and maximum comfort. Although your space should set a professional tone and have the requisite comforts you require, you may want to add a few personal touches—not only to buoy your sense of well-being but to offer a bit of yourself to others. Family photos, framed art, your diplomas, or a plant, perhaps, all offer nice touches. So do small collections of items from your professional work—books you've authored, awards, or pictures of you with colleagues at conferences. You should enjoy the space and make sure it works for you.

Now consider what you see. Are papers everywhere? Are files you haven't touched in years still lying in view? Could those empty cabinets hold archives that don't need to be a reach away?

If so, consider these tips:

- **Unclutter your desk.** Drawers are for items you don't use every day, so purge what you can and tuck only what's necessary inside a drawer within easy reach. Toss duplicates and anything you no longer need, such as year-old periodicals, books that are outdated, or files that support old projects. The paper clutter that occupies the top layer of your desk can largely be eliminated given that almost everything today exists in electronic format.

  One organized hospital CEO puts all the papers on his desk away before leaving for the day, a habit he cultivated early on while working for a major in the US Army. The major had the rather nasty habit of sweeping papers left on his subordinates' desks at day's end into their trash cans or onto their desk chairs or the floor. Although the habit of an end-of-the-day paperless desk was force-fed by a demanding boss, the CEO maintains today that he's better for it because it forced him to deal with every paper on his desk and to get things done. He says it also ensures that he excavates through layers to be sure nothing has been buried or forgotten, and it enables him to make the next day's to-do list.
- **Unclutter your computer desktop.** By now, most people know that saving documents, e-mail attachments, photos, and articles onto one's computer desktop is

both a confusing and a technologically heretical way to work—and yet, most of us do it. An overabundance of desktop files clogs your visual field, creates issues with older and newer versions, and slows your machine down. Put electronic documents in file folders in a safe and appropriate place right away. If you do it correctly the first time, you won't need to drag and drop stuff onto your desktop that will only be ignored, become irritating, and slow your machine down.

- **Develop a good filing system.** Every job requires a seamless way to keep paper and electronic documents organized. Don't put this task off—as soon as you begin a job, figure out what you need to save, how you need to save it, where it should exist, and what the names of the folders (electronic and paper) ought to be. Position those used regularly close at hand—on your right, for example, if you're right-handed.

  - Keep file names obvious, and include dates if appropriate. If you give file folders vague and undescriptive names, such as "Jeff's file" or "2014 projects," you will forget what the files contain and never be able to retrieve the right information. Consider using major categories and subcategories— for example, "Surgery–New Surgeon," "Surgery–Staff Raises," and "Surgery–Equipment Needs."

  - Organize electronic files that need regular archiving by month, then by year. Having a "Done" file alongside your "Pending" file is sometimes prudent, especially for regular tasks.

  - If you have an administrative assistant, consider using paper folders with each day's items organized according to the day of the week.

  - If you have direct reports and meet with them regularly, have a paper file for each individual, and drop in notes as they occur to you so that you can bring them up for discussion at your next meeting.

– To deal with some of the barrage of mail and paperwork that comes your way, have a reading file that contains nonurgent information that you can review while waiting for a flight, taking a taxi, or sitting on the train.

– If you need to retain files for a designated period, be sure to mark them with destruction dates. Most healthcare organizations have policies on retention of records, but destruction dates are easily and often overlooked.

– Keep a paper file on your own accomplishments, dropping in information as you go on what you've done, what impact it's had, how you've been recognized, and so on. Many companies require employees at all levels to complete a self-assessment and detail their accomplishments prior to their annual review, and keeping a personal file is a great way to have perfect recall when you complete this task or update your résumé.

– Above all, be sure to maintain the filing system you develop—because a system is only as good as its owner.

• **Keep priorities and to-do lists visible.** Update them often. Whether in a paper list or an electronic document, keep your top three to five priorities for the day close to your visual field. "Out of sight, out of mind" applies here: Visual reminders—and they can be simple—keep you on task, and it's always satisfying to check off what you've accomplished before moving on to what's next.

• **Know who's doing what.** For bigger projects, keep a record of what you have delegated to whom, and when it's due. Tickler files—such as a note on your calendar to follow up on something or a jotted-down due date with a "soft" deadline a week or so in advance of the "hard" deadline—are useful for keeping track of this information.

- **Have a way to keep track of ideas you have while on the go.** If you have a mobile device, use it to take notes if you're somewhere where a pen, paper, or computer is not available. Keep a pen and paper near your bed and in your car, and use them whenever ideas occur to you for projects. Schedule a regular time to retrieve these ideas and notes—the beginning and end of the day tend to be good—to keep tally of your thoughts and what needs to be accomplished.

- **Keep private things private.** Others who meet with you in your office may be able to see documents and messages on your computer screen that they really shouldn't be privy to. Therefore, consider using a screen to protect the privacy of your documents. Alternatively, you could also simply ensure your computer screen is always turned away from the direct view of your guests.

- **Conquer your calendar.** Rather than keep separate calendars at work and home, integrate the two. If you use the calendar on your mobile device, it will always be close at hand. Add standing meetings, important dates, birthdays, anniversaries, and annual conferences as recurring events so that they populate automatically.

- **Keep charged.** You need three cords to keep your mobile device charged. Have two cords for regular electrical outlets—one at home and one in the office. The third cord is a special charging apparatus that connects to the cigarette lighter in your car. Keep each cord where it belongs. Two at home and one in the car won't do you a lick of good if you're in your office.

- **Follow daily rituals.** Schedule time each day for reading and returning e-mails, returning phone calls, and making rounds, and limit yourself to the times scheduled. Be sure to build in time for traveling to meetings and to schedule extra time in case traffic is bad, meetings run long, or you need to stop for gas. Be sure to schedule at least one hour a day to take care of work at your desk so that you can reorient yourself to your priorities and prepare for upcoming deadlines and meetings.

- **End each day by prepping for the following one.** End-of-day rituals should include clearing your desk, putting things back in their places, and reviewing your calendar for the next day.

The effort you put into creating and maintaining an efficient work space will pay off hugely if you simply make sure to follow the structure you've set up. Instead of spending time and energy looking for things and moving piles from one area to the next, you'll be able to focus on productivity—and enjoy the space you've created.

EXERCISE 1

Examine your system for organizing electronic files on your computer. What are you doing well? What could you do better?

EXERCISE 2

Schedule a time to de-clutter your office. Recycle books, shred documents, and either file papers or discard them. Plan to do this at least annually.

RESOURCE

Online Business Buddy. 2013. *Organize Your Office: The Ultimate Guide to Organizing Your Office and Having a Stress-Free Workplace.* Kindle edition. Amazon Digital Services, Inc.

Identify and Support Culture

Success and professional satisfaction are greatly impacted by the culture of an organization and one's level of connection to it. Gaining the insight and perspective of key stakeholders within an organization is a critical and important step as you determine whether you will be a strong cultural fit.

—*Matt Mendez, MHA,*
senior consultant, Stroudwater Associates,
Wilmington, North Carolina

THINK ABOUT THE best job you've ever had. Then consider the reasons it was the best. Ten to one, it had something to do with the feel of the place—that difficult-to-pin-down warmth and collegiality of peers, the drive and vision of your supervisors, the fun you had tackling work challenges independently and in groups, and the satisfaction of finding solutions to the problems at hand. That *je ne sais quoi* is workplace culture.

But what goes into a company's culture—its feel—isn't so easy to pin down. Managers have something to do with it, as do a company's mission, vision, and goals. Employees play a large part, too.

One of the most rewarding routes to success is to have a hand in nurturing a great workplace culture. In healthcare, given the nobility of purpose—health, wellness, and stellar patient care, for starters—you've got a natural leg up on developing a positive culture because, at base, the field centers on helping people. But as a healthcare executive, you're responsible for filling in the rest and making your organization one that people will love, work hard in, and feel great loyalty to.

Do whatever you can to cultivate a place where employees are happy, loyal, and engaged and where they feel empowered to make a positive contribution. As you advance in your career and take on greater leadership roles and responsibilities, you will increasingly have opportunities to guide an organization's culture—but early on in your career, you can make a real mark by making your company a place people feel welcome in and loyal to and where they *want* to come to work.

We've all seen organizations where the employees are happy and work hard to make the company successful. These companies have a great workplace culture. So how did they get there?

- **Strong leadership.** A leader sets expectations and creates an environment where staffers carry out the company's values in clear, coherent, and visible fashion by fulfilling clearly laid-out goals. But not even the best leaders can constantly monitor staffers' behaviors and practices day in and day out. When peers hold one another accountable to organizational values and standards, a workplace culture is strong. And when people see their colleagues treating patients with care and respect, picking up the phone on the first ring, holding doors open, and greeting colleagues politely in the corridor, they can feel the tide of positivity and pride in their organization. There is buy-in. But how do you get there?

- **Agency and ownership.** Staff must have a say in the values and standards that a company puts in place. Frontline staff who interact directly with patients will embrace values and standards if they helped shape and define those measures as part of a formalized, thoughtful process. You don't want your employees to feel they're simply doing a job, clocking in and then clocking out. You want them to feel they are stakeholders in a positive, well-vetted vision and to enjoy long, meaningful careers with the company.

- **A bottom-up approach.** Although a strong leader drives an organization's mission, vision, and goals, a company's culture really takes hold when it has buy-in from the population of workers. Therefore, culture cannot be driven from the top down. To be a useful and powerful management tool, culture must be implemented through employee belief and participation.

When beginning your professional career, you'll want to find an organization that has a culture in which you'll thrive—a place where you'll feel in sync with the people, energy, mission, and momentum. You'll want to seek out a place that values participation, fosters creativity, and recognizes and rewards the motivated, determined, and smart. Given that you'll likely adopt the management style and culture of the places that provided flavor early on in your career, you should begin your professional life working for good role models, people you admire and want to emulate. Your first job (or your first two or three) should therefore be well and thoughtfully chosen, in tune with your work ethos and talents, and—if at all possible—as close to your dream environment as you can get.

If choosing those early jobs carefully is so important, how do you discern the corporate culture of an organization you're considering joining? A lot is evident just by looking around. As you tread through the parking lot and enter the buildings, what do you see? Do employees scurry around with their eyes cast down, or do they look up and smile? Do they look you in the eye, and are they genuinely helpful? Do you see people wasting time, huddled together in corners, or do they appear purposeful and busy? Is everyone new, are there boatloads of temporary workers, or do you meet veteran employees with tenure and perspective? Those are all clues.

Another way to glean information about a company's culture is to review its mission statement and compare it with what you see.

Who are the company's owners and leaders? When you meet with them, do they know and embody their own mission statements? Is the mission statement succinct and easy to remember?

Before you take a job at any organization, try to imagine how you'll fit in and whether you're a good match for the place. Do people dress formally, or is it more casual? Are the job descriptions well laid out and organized, or are the expectations nebulous and vague? Do you feel clear about the job's parameters after you've asked? Will there be an orientation? And are mentors available who can ease you into your role at the company?

Keep the following tactics in mind:

- **Cultivate and leverage your professional network.** Seek out people who work in organizations that interest you to gain their perspective. You likely already know someone (or an acquaintance has a connection) there, and online tools such as LinkedIn offer another route to identifying and networking with people in companies that interest you.
- **Gain the perspective of the general public.** Ask people how an organization that interests you is regarded within the community.
- **Conduct online research and media searches.** Online local news outlets and media coverage can provide excellent insight into an organization's culture and priorities and the public's opinion of it. How does it handle negative publicity? How accessible and well-spoken are its leaders? What problems and successes does it appear to have?

EXERCISE 1

Write a paragraph describing your company's culture. Identify its mission, vision, and goals. How does the culture of the organization affect the employees' work?

EXERCISE 2

Create a personal mission statement and detail what your values are. Compare and contrast your personal mission and values with those of organizations of interest to gauge your compatibility.

EXERCISE 3

Using the informational interview (see Lesson 38 on learning from others' careers), meet people who have been successful in leading companies with a workplace culture you feel is strong. Ask them what's special about their organization, how they make it special, and what they consider to be the top five ingredients in creating a positive culture. Study their approach by mapping out the route they took in establishing a strong workplace culture.

RESOURCES

American College of Healthcare Executives. 2011. "Creating an Ethical Culture Within the Healthcare Organization." Ethical policy statement. Revised November. www.ache.org/policy /environ.cfm.

Lindsey, J. S., and J. W. Mitchell. 2011. *Great Workplace Culture: The Supreme Competitive Advantage.* Ivy Ventures LLC white paper. www.box.net/shared/6nig8gky1i.

McKinnon, T. 2013. "How to Build a Great Company Culture." *Forbes.* Posted October 4. www.forbes.com/sites/groupthink /2013/10/04/how-to-build-a-great-company-culture/.

Patrick, J. 2013. "The Real Meaning of Corporate Culture." *The New York Times* Blog. Posted May 21. http://boss.blogs .nytimes.com/2013/05/21/the-real-meaning-of-corporate -culture/?_php=true&_type=blogs&_r=0.

Improve Quality and Safety

Safety is more important and more central than most people think. Paul O'Neill, a corporate leader, Secretary of the Treasury, and later healthcare leader in Pittsburgh, rebuilt a major world company, Alcoa, and moved it to market dominance. He did it using safety as the company-wide focus. Days of work lost from accidents became the metric for all the company's aluminum production and manufacturing. Over his 12 years as chair and CEO, the number was pushed down and down. With the decline, profits went up. Why? Because to build a safe workplace, you must study and improve work processes. The same is true in healthcare, twice over. Safe patient care is cheaper and more effective, and it generates higher HCAHPS scores. A safe work environment cuts labor costs, reduces lost time, and builds loyalty.

—*John R. Griffith, MBA, LFACHE,*
professor emeritus, Department of Health Management & Policy,
University of Michigan School of Public Health, Ann Arbor

YOUR MOST IMPORTANT job as a healthcare executive is to ensure the safety of patients, employees, and visitors—essentially everyone who enters your organization's work environment. Immediate correction of threats to quality and safety comes before any other priority. Work on the organization's goals, vision, and long-term strategy cannot proceed until everyone is safe.

The day when patient safety and quality were solely the purview of the physician has passed. Today's healthcare executives need to be conversant in medical terminology, understand the basics of procedures and machinery, and know something about disease management and care delivery processes to have a solid perspective and understanding of the route to the best, safest, and highest-quality care. They must comprehend how to improve, step by step, the quality of care given to all patients and how to ensure that safety remains paramount in an organization's ethos. Because you will likely be held increasingly responsible not only for your hospital's financial outcomes but for its clinical ones as well, taking an active role in understanding processes and procedures is a solid first step toward asserting your commitment to the place and its people.

Consider the following points as you prepare for executive responsibility:

- **Know what it means.** Knowing medical lingo and a bit of biology isn't enough. To become an expert, you will also need to study quality and safety as a subject matter topic, reading case studies that describe what kinds of initiatives have worked well for organizations of a particular type and size—and which attempts at improvement have failed, and why. Take time to understand the relevant terminology as you do your research. You should be able to read and understand the quality and safety indicators that are driven by the Centers for Medicare & Medicaid Services and various third-party contracts and agreements. If you are working in a hospital or other provider institution, there is likely a series of documents that explicitly state how quality and safety are practiced and measured—find them, and pore over them. The more you read, the more you'll know. Absorb everything you can in this area.

- **Develop a culture of improvement.** As you work to make things better, involve everyone—from the board of trustees on down. Talk about what you think might need work in the areas of quality and safety, and listen intently to what others believe are areas of strength and deficit in this regard. Be open and honest about your organization's shortcomings, and join your colleagues in seeking solutions. Ingrain the importance of specific, tangible, visible programs—for example, nurses might wear a fluorescent sash as a sign of concentration as they measure outpatient medications so that others don't interrupt them—and, as new ideas take root, talk about how a particular initiative is going. Express your continued reliance on your colleagues, and remind them repeatedly that an open, communicative culture is the best first step toward making thoughtful, prudent, lasting change.

- **Express quality and safety in financial terms.** In addition to being the right thing to do, doing something right the first time is always most cost-effective. Preventable errors can lead to everything from a poor organizational reputation for quality to fines, bad press, and lawsuits. Let your colleagues and employees understand the financial fallout from errors in a dollars-and-cents manner by giving them examples. For example, *Each of the ____ hospital-acquired infections at one local medical center cost it more than $____ million. Unnecessary duplication of medical procedures cost the patient $____ as well as untold wasted hours and stress.* Institutions follow their quality indicators closely because payments from federal, state, and various third-party sources are increasingly based on quality and safety. Quality and safety matter for myriad reasons—including the bottom line. Express it as such.

- **Look for sustainable, systematic solutions to problems.** Stop the immediate threat, of course, before changing the system so that the threat does not recur. Take care not to overcomplicate it—sometimes the best solutions are simple, inexpensive, and easy to implement. Got a hand-washing compliance problem? Place signage outside and inside the room, along with sinks and soap. Encourage patients to ask nurses and physicians whether they've washed their hands. Institute "undercover" hand-hygiene observers to monitor compliance at random times.

- **Measure and continually improve.** If patient falls appear to be on the rise on a particular unit, dig into the situation, determine the cause of the increase, and then improve the process to prevent future falls. Don't overlook simple solutions, though they may not always solve the entire problem. The solution may be simple, such as changing the brand of floor wax or the floor-cleaning schedule. Perhaps an increasing number of elderly patients are being treated in a particular wing of the hospital, or nursing staff have too high a patient load. Training in Lean and Six Sigma improvement methodologies may help solve safety and quality problems such as these.

- **Practice and measure.** A good plan is a key component of a successful safety program. Make yours as thoughtful and responsive to all facets of the problem as possible. As you develop your plan, make sure that it's current with best practices and continually followed up and improved on. Pay close attention to details as you examine an issue before determining a course of action. After you create a plan, monitor the issue and watch for improvements.

Thus, if your hospital has a growing problem with infections, it may stem from something as basic as poor hand washing or lackluster care of medical instruments. At the outset, you might ask what procedures and reminders are in place for hand-washing compliance and stethoscope cleaning. Then you might inquire about institutional benchmarks and look at the ways other organizations have solved similar issues to prevent infection. What changes can your organization make to improve your results? What are the hand-washing benchmarks? How will you measure whether you're moving the needle in a positive direction?

- **Report your results.** It's often said that what gets measured gets improved. Insist on transparency, even if the issue is a sensitive one. (*All* issues are likely sensitive, so you'd best be open about everything.) Share the shortcomings with your colleagues and employees—and tell them about the success that you hope procedural improvements will bring.

- **Develop the personal skills needed to improve safety and quality.** Ensure that both you yourself and the members of your team have the knowledge and skills you need to undertake improvements.

  - Familiarize yourself with the initiatives of the Institute for Healthcare Improvement (IHI).
  - Learn about Lean or Six Sigma improvement techniques.
  - Enhance your clinical understanding, especially if you don't have a nursing or medical background.
  - Support and work with interprofessional teams to identify opportunities for improvement.
  - Support regular training programs for all. Quality and safety are dependent on the best available evidence and successful practices. Continuing education programs—such as workshops, lectures, retreats, and professional development days—are essential for everyone.

Above all, develop a passion for improving quality and promoting safety throughout your career in healthcare. It is, after all, the most basic, fundamental way to help.

EXERCISE 1

Identify a process in your organization that needs improving, writing down what you observe. Is the intensive care unit rife with dissonant, impossible-to-locate patient alarms that fatigue the ears of staffers and patients? Are patients not sleeping in the labor and delivery unit because of door slamming and elevator chirps? Is the emergency room waiting area clogged with sick people who are backlogged for hours? Are reception staff overwhelmed and terse? Jot down a list of red flags. Try to identify some possible problems and their solutions.

EXERCISE 2

Earn an IHI Open School Basic Certificate of Completion in healthcare quality and safety.

RESOURCES

Institute for Healthcare Improvement (IHI). 2014. "Open School." Accessed November 11. www.ihi.org/education /ihiopenschool/Pages/default.aspx.

White, K. R., and J. R. Griffith. 2015. *The Well-Managed Healthcare Organization,* eighth edition, in press. Chicago: Health Administration Press.

Listen to Your Stakeholders

We tend to underestimate the symbolic meaning we carry
in our roles as leaders. Most people are surprised, pleased,
honored, or encouraged that we truly want to listen to them.
When visiting with any stakeholder, leave something behind,
such as a future appointment, a handwritten note on the
flyleaf of a small book, or even your business card with your
cell phone number handwritten on it. They will be grateful.

—*Kenneth D. Graham, FACHE,*
acting president, North Hawaii Community Hospital, Kamuela,
and 2011 recipient of the ACHE Gold Medal Award

IF HEALTHCARE ORGANIZATIONS aim to serve their communities with the best, highest-quality care, a manager's very first priority must be to determine what's working—and what's not. Those we serve—our patients, customers, stakeholders, clients, or whatever you choose to call them—hold the key to helping us understand where and how to improve and, ultimately, how to be more successful. Based on the answers they provide, it's up to the healthcare organization's managers to identify improvements so that the quality of connections within is exceptional, compassionate, and informed by the very best practices.

So what's the best way to find out what customers want? It's simple: Just ask. But figuring out whom to ask, and how, is less straightforward. Unlike a traditional business, which sells products or services to a particular constituent, healthcare delivery is complex, as is a healthcare organization's customer base. For-profit businesses fill their coffers by keeping customers happy to ensure they continue spending. Healthcare organizations, however, have a far nobler purpose: to make people and their communities healthier. And although the patient is a customer, so are a host of others.

Healthcare employees are stakeholders because they're the ones who provide the services as agents of the owners. Physicians are stakeholders because they choose where to refer their patients for healthcare. Insurance companies are stakeholders because they shop around for the best, most profitable provider contracts. Employers are stakeholders because they pay for the bulk of the costs related to their employees' health insurance. A host of stakeholders and decision makers must be considered in the mix—well before a customer ever presents himself as a patient.

Getting close to your customers in healthcare, then, means listening to everyone. So how, exactly, do you do that? Break it down. Begin with the three most important groups, as described below. As you connect with people within, touching, and outside your organization, consider these five steps to guide your interaction: Ask. Listen. Think. Care. Respond.

- **Patients and their families.** Talk to patients on your rounds. Introduce yourself, and ask open-ended questions such as "How are we doing?" Listen intently to what they say, taking notes and showing you care. If they offer specific complaints (rotten parking, complicated billing issues, inconvenient visiting hours), follow up with them to tell them how you solved their problems and concerns, if you have done so. If you can't solve their problems, let them know you've listened and are considering ways to make the services better. Leave them with a business card, genuine gratitude, and the sense that they've offered you something extremely important—which they have.

You may wish to cultivate a particular vein of conversation with patients and families, if you're looking for feedback on specific initiatives. Perhaps you'd ask questions such as the following:

— "We are proud of the compassionate care we offer here, and I wondered what you thought of it?"
— "If there was one thing that might have made your experience here more positive, what would it be? How would it benefit you?"
— "Have we made you feel safe and well cared for here? What specifics made the difference?"
— "Were there particular staffers who impressed you (and may I pass on the compliment)?"

• **Employees and volunteers.** Leaders and managers exist to solve problems so that employees on the front lines of a healthcare organization can do what they do best: offer the most compassionate, highest-quality patient-centered care they're capable of. These individuals occupy a critical role as they deliver small and large kindnesses that are remembered in ways that surgeons, specialists, and administrators often aren't recalled. Frontline staff are truly every healthcare organization's lifeblood, its foundation, and the key to extraordinary quality and service.

A successful patient-centered organization is also an employee-focused organization. Connect with your employees, take the time to get to know them, and respond to them. Employees who feel valued, listened to, well supported, and personally cared for will not only be immensely loyal to their organization; they'll also pay these kindnesses forward to their patients and their patients' families. A good way to start a dialogue with employees and volunteers on your rounds is to ask, "Do you have the tools you need to do your job?" Additional questions might include the following:

– "What bogs you down or gets in your way of doing your best?"

– "What are some of the concerns you hear from your patients about the hospital? What concerns do you perceive your colleagues have? What are your concerns?"

– "How can managers like me be of better service to you? What can we do to offer you a platform for even better performance?"

– "What's your favorite part of your job? Who are your favorite colleagues?"

– "What skills could you learn that would help you feel more competent and confident in your job?"

– "Are there other responsibilities or jobs here you'd like to be involved in?"

• **Other stakeholders.** Just as important as patients/families and employees/volunteers are the physicians who operate within and around your organization. You must make a herculean effort to stay close to your physicians (see Lesson 30 on engaging physician colleagues), listen to their needs and concerns, and respond competently, effectively, and promptly to those concerns. Other key stakeholders with whom you should conduct listening rounds include community leaders, referring physicians and provider organizations, and policymakers (including elected government representatives, from your city's mayor to your state and federal representatives and senators). Listen, as well, to members of the media, your organization's board, donors, suppliers, payers, and anyone else who is connected to or has a stake in your community's health and well-being.

- Get better at listening to this third catch-all group by means of the following:
  - Figure out how to have fewer meetings so that you can conduct rounds more often and thereby identify opportunities for improvement in real time.
  - Schedule time to meet customers. Make sure all the members of your team schedule time to meet with customers, too.
  - Include hospitality among your organization's values. Treat those who are part of your organization (or merely stepping across its threshold) as you would if they were special guests in your home. Make sure they feel both safe and welcome.
  - Arrange and participate in ongoing professional development for all stakeholders on resilience, collaboration, and sound communication techniques. (Topics to explore might include how to handle difficult conversations, how to be a better team player, or how to practice gentle yoga.) Provide incentives (food, professional development credit, free parking) to get people in the door, and require a level of participation from staff that is doable and not an encumbrance.
  - Learn all you can about "active listening," and then practice, practice, practice.

In healthcare, the only constant is change—so it's critical to notice what's really happening from *all* angles. Inexperienced managers commonly listen to one side's story and then start making changes without considering the effect of those changes on other departments or even on the organization's strategic focus.

Don't promise to fix something for someone until you get all the facts and the entire story—otherwise, you'll find yourself spinning your wheels and stirring up ire among groups you hadn't meant to affect.

The whole point of listening, of course, is to help your organization deliver on its mission more effectively. And although you won't be able to solve all the problems you encounter or give everyone every item on their wish lists, if you connect your decisions to your organization's vision, values, and goals you'll have been true to your role as a transformational leader. Opening lines of communication, gathering information, and then using that information to influence how decisions are made is as critical to an organization's success as its cash flow, operations, marketing, and strategic planning. Your role fuses the bottom line with your organization's heart.

EXERCISE 1

Set aside one hour three times a week to make rounds for the sole purpose of listening to patients, employees, physicians, and other stakeholders. Meet them where they are—on patient units, in the cafeteria, in the surgery lounge, or in their offices. Ask open-ended questions, taking notes as you listen intently to their answers, and identify ways—big and small—to improve operations and to make their jobs and lives easier.

EXERCISE 2

Read a book or take a course on active listening.

RESOURCES

Chapman, S. G. 2012. *The Five Keys to Mindful Communication: Using Deep Listening and Mindful Speech to Strengthen*

Relationships, Heal Conflicts, and Accomplish Your Goals. Boston: Shambhala Publications.

Freeman, R. E., J. S. Harrison, and A. C. Wicks. 2007. *Managing for Stakeholders: Survival, Reputation, and Success.* New Haven, CT: Yale University Press.

Hoppe, M. 2007. *Active Listening: Improve Your Ability to Listen and Lead.* Greensboro, NC: Center for Creative Leadership.

Manage Your Messaging

Managing messaging is one of the most important skill sets for both managers and leaders. Every day of the year, even before I leave for the office, I hop on the Internet and look for the important news and journal articles of the day. I pull and place the key ones I want to send in what I call "Market News" to hundreds of managers, physicians, and staff members throughout my organization. This connects me to them daily, gives them information I think is important, and helps to set the context for the changes ahead. And because the articles are not written by me or my organization, they are received more objectively. This is just one example of messaging, or "teaching," that is also a critical role of a manager.

—Chris Van Gorder, FACHE,
president and CEO, Scripps Health System,
San Diego, California

A GIFTED FORMER student was a top achiever in our executive health administration program, and as a nurse manager she had a lot of potential to advance professionally into more senior-level positions. What held her back, she confided, was her inability to communicate well and to think, as she described it, "on her feet."

She wasn't being modest or self-deprecating. Her deficit went well beyond a fear of public speaking—she lacked the confidence, organization, and quality control to offer strong, succinct messages to her audiences. She couldn't articulate quickly, convey her meaning well, or express herself in a manner that rallied and inspired her colleagues.

Fast-forward 15 years, however, and she had become a hospital CEO who appeared often in TV news interviews with poise, expressive body language, and an engaging pitch and tone. But in addition to these superficial aspects of communication style, she had the ability to send clear, concise, and understandable messages that were appropriately geared to her audience. So what had happened? Plain and simple: She had worked on her messaging skills, simplified and honed her messages, studied best practices—and improved dramatically.

Some people are naturals at sending meaningful, articulate, eloquent, and well-crafted messages, always knowing what to say and how to say it. They understand and use messaging to get power, exert influence, and obtain leverage. The rest of us? We have to practice, as the former student did, to make our messaging stronger.

To succeed as a manager, of course, you have to communicate effectively. When you're in a management or leadership position, others look to you for direction, for inspiration, and for information. And obviously it's not only *what* you say, but *how* you say it. Whether the audience is a small group of clinicians or the entire staff of a huge medical center, a leader's messages must be consistent, clear, and well thought out as well as connected to the organization's mission, vision, and values.

Micromessaging refers to how a message is tailored to a particular audience. When speaking to a small team or work group, for example, you may offer the same overarching message as you would to the entire establishment, but with a different nuance or texture. You'd address people by name, add humor (but only if you're actually good at it), and perhaps weave in stories and anecdotes about some of those present to ally yourself with the group and cultivate a feeling of intimacy.

That kind of intimacy is important. Even when conveying information about financial performance or sharing statistics and quality measures, you need—in healthcare especially—to connect your messages to the humans who keep the place humming and whose efforts in safety, quality, and compassion lie at the very heart of the organization's success. Many smart senior healthcare leaders aren't able to connect their messages to their stakeholders and therefore lose their audience's attention—and their regard. Although you may be terrific at sharing news about, say, a financial turnaround, if you fail to mention what's at the core of it—the people—you're sure to lose your colleagues' loyalty and to tarnish your reputation. Employees, physicians, nurses, and board members want to know that their leader understands the connection between their decisions and outcomes and the organization's mission, vision, and values. Some people are so good at such messaging that they achieve lofty career heights even without positive statistical trends to back them.

As a healthcare leader, you can learn to manage your messaging more effectively through simple planning and practice. Here are some tips:

- **Choose the medium.** The most persuasive messages are delivered in person. Telephone, e-mail, and text messages are less persuasive ways to communicate and often result in misunderstandings of tone, aim, and content.

- **Master your delivery.** How you say it is just as important as what you say. Although you don't have to be a stage performer to be a good speaker, your personal commitment and passion about the subject matter should sing through your message. Speak with authority, clarity, and confidence. Be eloquent, but speak plainly enough to ensure you're understood. Use voice tone, inflection, and pitch to your advantage, and enunciate clearly and use enough pauses to ensure your audience stays with you, particularly if you're sharing dense information.

- **Tell the truth.** People appreciate being leveled with, so if you're sharing bad news, be up front, factual, and frank about it, and then move on to solutions. Keep your messages congruent with your values. If you compromise your core beliefs to manipulate an outcome, others will pick up on your insincerity.

- **Be brief.** Group key points into buckets. If your purpose is to share information, offer facts with an anecdote illustrating each point so that it's more easily remembered. Keep your buckets to a maximum of three.

- **Avoid jargon.** Don't overuse acronyms, medical-speak, or technical jargon. Use simple words and simple sentences, but without being overly casual. Don't address your audience as "you guys" or talk the way you did in college; keep your words professional.

- **Monitor your body language.** Keep your facial expression in sync with the tone and content of your message. Bad news should not be delivered with a smirk or smile, and good tidings should not involve a sour or expressionless face. Especially if your message is being recorded, your gestures should be confined to the area near your waist and not distract from your face. Your gaze should be steady but not staring.

- **Know your talking points.** Don't lose your message in the medium or dart off down tangential rabbit trails at the slightest provocation. Stay on point. Be consistent and convincing in your position, state it firmly and clearly, and know when to stop. News reporters will take advantage if they sense you're waffling or easily distracted.

- **Know your audience.** Although your talking points may essentially be the same whether you're addressing a large group or a small one, you should tailor your message to the audience. Put yourself in their place. What are their particular concerns about or interests in the topic? If you're talking about your new accountable care organization, for example, you'd address an audience of physicians very differently than you would a board of directors or community forum. Be respectful of people's time and understanding—tailor what you say.

- **Understand you'll have critics.** Some people will take what you say out of context and attempt to use your message against you. Don't let these individuals fluster or anger you; manage the situation by remembering your main points and refusing to engage in a tangential discussion that puts you on the defensive. Know when to stop talking, and if questions persist, say firmly, "I believe I've answered your question—I don't think I can say more. Let's move on."

As a healthcare leader, you'll need to communicate regularly with your key stakeholders about the organization's health, the issues it faces, its progress on overarching goals, and any major decisions that will affect everyone. Although you will share similar messages over and over again, with the same talking points, remember that to many people the information is brand-new—so treat every message as though you're giving your talk for the first time. Even if you feel you're "hypercommunicating," your message will be well received if it is well thought out and delivered succinctly, truthfully, and in an organized fashion.

EXERCISE 1

If proper messaging is holding back your career, hire a communications coach.

EXERCISE 2

The best teacher is the camera, so ask a reporter or journalist to help you practice being interviewed in front of a camera, take a media training class, or find a continuing education program to help you improve your communication skills.

RESOURCE

Young, S. 2006. *Micromessaging: Why Great Leadership Is Beyond Words.* New York: McGraw-Hill.

Raise Your Hand Boldly

Complete small responsibilities and projects with the same enthusiasm and leadership as the perceived "significant" ones. The truth is that all tasks are important and present valuable learning experiences. Not one of us is above any of them.

Just this summer, one of our administrative interns had the assignment to evaluate how mail was currently being delivered and to make recommendations. The project really wasn't about the mail at all, but how to influence and make recommendations in an area that you do not have any knowledge of and how to engage the staff to help in the solutions. That is a skill that can be applied to any situation.

—Terrie Edwards, MHA, FACHE,
president, Sentara Leigh Hospital,
Norfolk, Virginia

IMAGINE IT: YOUR CEO says at a team meeting, "We need volunteers to work on a project to improve patient flow in the emergency department." Patient flow is not your area of expertise, your office is several buildings away from the emergency department, and you don't even know the name of anyone who works there. So what do you do?

Raise your hand!

Volunteering for projects in disparate parts of your organization can help you gain experience and learn new skills. It can enable you to interface with a whole new group of colleagues you may not otherwise see. And if you develop a reputation as someone who can identify problems and solutions and work hard to get things done outside the confines of your job description, you'll not only be appreciated—you'll be noticed.

Why volunteer for projects?

- **Volunteering can expose you to new areas of your organization.** Young professionals often find themselves in jobs with narrow scopes, which can lead to organizational tunnel vision and the erroneous sense that tasks that fall outside the parameters of one's job description cannot be touched. Don't be deceived by such notions.

- **Volunteering expands your vantage.** Volunteering is a great way to understand the larger issues confronting your organization. Working on company-wide projects and initiatives will also help you see how everything is interrelated. With this knowledge, you will be better prepared to take jobs with more responsibility in the future.

- **Volunteer projects are a great way to network and meet new people.** Working on projects outside your usual domain will enable you to meet new people throughout your organization. Establishing a far-reaching network is a good way to solve problems and to tap broad resources when you tackle issues down the road. It can also introduce you to distant allies who may be able to help you bypass more cumbersome routes to quickly obtain the information or results you're after.

- **Volunteering helps you grow your gifts and develop new skills.** Want to develop stronger leadership skills? Volunteer to be an officer of a social or volunteer organization such as Habitat for Humanity or United Way. Not only will you develop a wide variety of contacts outside your company, you'll also have a chance to interface professionally with other like-minded individuals and to hone your skills as a speaker, a professional, and a go-to person. And besides advancing the common good, you'll spread the message that such values are important to you and your organization.

- **Volunteering will earn you a reputation as someone who gets things done and isn't afraid of work.** Show you're not too big a snob to roll up your sleeves and pitch in. Develop a personal brand as someone who can work on a project and get effective results, someone who can take a problem—however big or small—and solve it. Don't shirk from menial tasks, should they come up—get in there and tackle them with grace, good humor, and respect for those who do such tasks every day.

And don't always wait to be asked to help—step up!

Perhaps your organization is struggling with declining revenue and volume, a problem you've been mulling over. At a leaders' meeting at which the problem is being discussed, you might say, "I think we should consider focusing our efforts on working more closely with our physicians to find out how we can make it easier for them to bring patients to our hospital."

You might go on to share, "Several physicians and patients have recently mentioned to me the difficulties they face when trying to schedule procedures at our outpatient center. I'd love the chance to lead a team to look into and solve this problem, to see if perhaps a solution can be determined that would help grow volume for our hospital."

Would you like to learn more about your organization's information technology systems? Volunteer to become your department's expert on their use, or ask to be included in its system users' group. With a little effort, you can become the go-to person when computer problems arise. This is an example of identifying a problem and generating your own role in helping solve it, for both yourself and others.

Is your organization raising money for a local charity? Participating in fundraising efforts is a great way to meet people in your organization over a good cause. Holiday charity drives for food, toys, or financial assistance are a great way to help, show leadership, and join your colleagues in togetherness.

If your employer does not offer opportunities for strengthening your financial skills, consider becoming the treasurer of a local charity to achieve that goal. Basic accounting functions are much the same from organization to organization, and you'll be able to better understand the healthcare business by working on real problems in real organizations.

Organizations are always looking for people who want to join problem-solving teams, and volunteering is an excellent way to work on projects outside your comfort zone and to interface professionally with people whom you would not otherwise encounter. Don't be that person who only raises his hand when the CEO is giving away free tickets to the basketball game. If you work hard and share your talents with people, departments, and organizations that need them, perhaps one day it'll be your box seats at the basketball game that will be up for grabs!

EXERCISE 1

Identify a social service organization that personally interests you, and ask the staff there how you might be of service. Volunteer your time for a single day or for a single project—such as United Way's Day of Caring—or offer your skills as part of a committee or on a more regular basis. Compile a journal to help you comprehend and maximize the value of the project to your career development, keeping a running tally of your contributions. Remember to thank the organizer of your project for allowing you to contribute.

EXERCISE 2

Make time in your schedule to meet with people interested in health administration as a career. Or plant seeds for future interest in health administration by volunteering to speak at a local high school or college about the various health profession careers.

RESOURCES

Corporation for National & Community Service. www.national service.gov.

VolunteerMatch. www.volunteermatch.org.

Defuse Generational Conflicts

As a senior healthcare executive, I've had the opportunity to work in many different organizations and have reported to individuals both older and younger than I, or with more or less experience than I had. No matter the circumstances, though, I've used every situation to learn and grow as a leader and as a colleague, and to apply these learnings for the benefit of the organization's mission.

—Jerrold Maki, MHA, FACHE,
vice president, Stanford Medical Center,
Palo Alto, California

THE LOGICAL CONSEQUENCE of Americans living and working longer than ever before reveals itself in the mishmash of ages in any given workplace. Baby boomers, Gen Xers, millennials, and others arrive at their jobs informed by a variety of experiences, expectations, and interpersonal styles—and with effort all around, they can work together seamlessly, respectfully, and harmoniously. But that tone of respect is set by their leader. When leaders learn to see and appreciate the value in everyone present, whether they are of the same age and generation or not, they bring out the best in people and enable the village—the team—to perform well, thoughtfully, and cohesively.

Here are a few pointers for those who work with colleagues of different ages and from a variety of backgrounds (which, frankly, is pretty much all of us):

- **Learn to accept help wherever you find it.** Those just starting out sometimes tend to think they have all the answers. But with growing wisdom, age, and experience comes an often gradual realization that we *all* need help and can't go it alone. One sign of a confident, competent leader is the ability to listen to advice from those who wish to give it, whether they're older, younger, less educated, more senior, or otherwise. You will begin to grow as a leader when you realize that you do not have all the answers and you start seeking advice from your colleagues—and not just your top brass—and listen earnestly to what they say. Two (or three or four) are better than one.

- **Expand beyond your peers.** Be open to and warm with everyone on your team—not just those whom you'd prefer to have lunch with or who are more in line with your age, political views, or social class. Exchange pleasantries and chitchat with all team members, making sure never to play favorites or to be cliquish such that some people or groups feel left out or excluded.

- **Be respectful.** Do you cringe when you hear, "Back in *my* day, it wasn't so easy, and we used to. . ."? Cringe-worthy or not, all employees—especially older workers who have been around longer—deserve to be listened to and have their points of view respected. Health systems have changed dramatically in recent years, and these individuals climbed the ranks in a different world where progression up the career ladder was more predictable and took place over the course of years. Respect their contributions and history, and understand that the job you have today exists because of past structures and the support and contributions of earlier generations.

- **Do you work to live, or live to work?** Everyone approaches this issue differently. Some expect their jobs to finish at 5 p.m. and not resume until 9 a.m. the next morning, no matter the circumstance or time of year, whereas others are in constant contact by phone, e-mail, or text. Whatever the viewpoint, drive your employees fairly while they're on task in the office, keeping your expectations high but manageable, and remember to be respectful of their off-hours when people leave for the day. Not everyone is driven by a 24/7 mentality of über-connectedness and will resent the implication that they're slacking off if they're not constantly accessible.

- **Ditch the notion of a perfect job, employee, or organization.** Young workers with limited work experience (other than an internship or two) often expect products to be flawless and processes to always make sense. Such expectations are not only unrealistic, they're untenable—and they can be irritating or degrading to other, more seasoned employees who have seen people come and go. Don't expect perfection, and know that the jobs you do won't be perfect either—and that's fine. With time and experience, you'll understand that *all* jobs and companies have problems that may be exasperating if they're not addressed efficiently. You'll learn a great deal about the healthcare business if you stay and work through problems rather than throw your hands up in frustration every time you run into an obstacle.

- **Be realistic about your abilities.** Just because you received a master's degree from a prestigious university doesn't mean you have all the answers. Many of the best CEOs got their skills from real-world—not textbook—experiences and through a lot of listening and collaborating with others. If a solution seems easy to you, you'd be wise to discuss it with some of your older colleagues first because it has likely been attempted before. You may learn some valuable information or history about the organization that will inform the answers you propose so that they'll *really* work—because they're guided by a longer-term perspective.

- **Have realistic expectations.** While it's great to imagine a Mark Zuckerberg brand of near-instant success, such achievements are exceedingly rare. Most of us have to pay our dues in terms of education and experience to make progress in our careers. So although you likely won't swoop in and improve patient care, increase clinician retention, and dramatically boost your hospital's bottom line all in the first six months through your own brand of personal dynamism, slow, steady, meaningful progress is within your reach if you work hard, include others, and set reasonable expectations for yourself. Having a realistic view of the healthcare world, your abilities, and the manner in which you will climb the corporate ladder is essential.

- **Don't be a job hopper.** Think about your brand *before* you decide to change jobs. If you switch jobs or industries every year or two, how will it look on your résumé? Gaps or quick moves from position to position can make you look flighty, unfocused, and unreliable. Appearing to be a job hopper is not to your advantage, and during interviews you may be asked to explain it. How long you stay at a place matters. Plan to stay at every job for at least five years. Give every job your best shot, and if it's not a good fit, make sure you're leaving for something better and for the right reasons. If you change positions every time you're confronted with a problem, experience conflict with a coworker, or find your interest and attention wilting, refocus yourself with purpose. Those who stay on to tackle difficult problems—and such problems exist in every job—will glean far more than will those who skedaddle every time the going gets tough.

EXERCISE 1

Invite one of your older, more seasoned colleagues to lunch or coffee. Ask her opinion about how to proceed with some of the problems you're working on, and show that you value her insight.

EXERCISE 2

When tackling your next problem or project, seek advice and counsel from a wider group of people than you would normally use—perhaps double the usual number. Try tapping people other than your usual suspects and including people of different ages. See what comes of this experiment, and take note of any staff strengths you hadn't anticipated.

RESOURCE

Taylor, P., and Pew Research Center. 2014. *The Next America: Boomers, Millennials, and the Looming Generational Showdown.* New York: PublicAffairs.

Manage Your Boss

One of the greatest lessons I ever learned was how important it was to manage my boss. Knee-deep in a successful career, having already led two hospitals as chief nurse, my third chief-of-nursing role offered a wake-up call that I needed to be better at "managing up." Our organization embarked on a 360-degree assessment of all executives, and I was rated exemplary by everyone but one person: my boss. After picking myself up off the floor, I found that my autonomous style wasn't enough. That concept of "managing up" helped me understand the importance of keeping my boss informed, sharing vision and goals, and developing effective two-way communication. Today, I use what I learned to coach new leaders. And while it sounds simple, it's most often communication basics that get in the way of true success.

—Shirley Gibson, DNP, MSHA, RN, FACHE,
associate vice president of nursing,
Virginia Commonwealth University Health System,
Richmond

BOSSES COME IN all varieties, from overbearing to absent, intrusive to inspiring—and in most cases, you can't control that. But you *can* control how competent, cooperative, reliable, and honest *you* are. You depend on your boss to give you what you need to work well and to explain how you are connected to the larger purposes and goals of your organization. You both need a relationship that's built on mutual respect and regular communication. And a prerequisite is having a realistic view of one another's abilities, weaknesses, implicit and explicit goals, work style, and needs—all informed by an ongoing level of respect and openness.

The most important work relationship for you to manage is the one with your boss. If you're not working hard at it, you're likely not as motivated or engaged as you should be. Managing your boss well—and being manageable yourself—enables you to do your best, to identify and own your success, and to benefit yourself and your organization in the process.

As the employee, you must learn how your boss processes information and makes decisions, what she expects from you, and the best way to negotiate priorities. What works with one boss may not work with another, so early on in your job you should assess how you can work together to manage expectations, understand your roles and responsibilities, and maximize your results. Figure out which ways you'll be best heard—and which tactics will get you a vacant, glassy-eyed stare as you talk. Employee–boss relationships can be maddening, but by offering your best work and a dogged determination to respectfully connect and engage, you'll be doing your part to build a successful relationship.

It is, however, a two-way street, and a successful working relationship can mean great results.

One boss—we'll call her Anne—was brought in to take over a newly restructured division of marketing and business development at a midsized hospital. Although Anne had significant experience in marketing—she had founded and sold an advertising agency prior to her arrival—she lacked experience with large, unwieldy organizations and nonprofits. Anne certainly had the competence for the task, which was to increase market share, but she lacked real experience with larger, more corporate-minded organizational operations. However, her second-in-command had what she didn't have, and together they complemented one another beautifully. Both were open about their own strengths and deficits, and both routinely reminded their staff that they depended on one another—and their larger team—to achieve the kind of results that were win–win all around.

Whether you're aiming to cultivate a strong, respectful relationship with your boss or hoping to become the best boss you can be, keep these ideas in mind:

- **Know what's expected.** Managing expectations is key to knowing how to focus your time and energy. Without clarity, you and your supervisor or employee may be working out of sync. Always ask, clarify, and check in. You might ask, "What does 'good' look like on this project?" or "If this went exactly the way you wanted it to go, turning out perfectly, what would happen between now and the end of the project?" It is your job to coax these important answers out of your boss, especially if he doesn't offer explanations first, or freely. Clarify your role by questioning, checking in, and then repeating those steps until the project is completed.

- **Understand your boss's perspective and adjust your approach.** Business guru Peter Drucker notes two key leadership communication styles: readers and listeners. Examine your boss's style, determine whether she prefers to receive information orally or in print, and tailor your communications accordingly. Also, determine whether your boss takes the long view or immediately jumps on the available facts.

- **Provide information at your boss's comfort level.** Although you are not a mind reader, you may sometimes have to guess what your boss needs or wants. Your boss may forget to tell you details that could save you time. Take the initiative to learn as much as you can about every new project you're assigned. Be up front about deadlines, resources, and point people at a project's outset. If a project isn't going as expected, let your boss know, and don't sugarcoat issues to please because your boss wants honesty. Always consider timing, which affects one's ability to be heard. Don't approach your boss to discuss a problem when he is preoccupied, stressed, or working under a tight deadline. If you're tuned in to him, you'll know when the right time is.

- **Be open if there has been a miscommunication.** Your boss is in charge, but that doesn't mean that you should be a yes-man. If you disagree with your boss, say so—but do it respectfully, and be prepared to back up what you say with facts and a well-rehearsed (and firm but gentle) argument. Begin your statements with "I think" or "I feel" so you own your points of view and feelings. For example, after an uncomfortable or confrontational dialogue, you might say, "I need to check in with you about our conversation yesterday. When you expressed what you did, I felt hurt and upset. Is that what you meant? Did I misunderstand?" It's up to you to say you don't fully understand what transpired. Similarly, it's your responsibility to speak up when you feel or think you haven't been heard.

- **Respect your boss and her position.** If you have bad news to impart, tell your boss first—no surprises, no undermining her in front of others, no one-upmanship. When you present a problem, be prepared to offer solutions rather than making your boss shoulder it entirely. And on a practical level, when you're new, don't regularly arrive later than or leave before your boss does. You not only want to be accessible and open to dialogue in those early days; you also want to show you're working hard and to the best of your ability—and that you're around and able to help.

- **Seek feedback on your performance.** Though you don't want to seem "high maintenance" or constantly self-centered, asking your boss for occasional feedback is important as you settle into a position. If your boss offers only positive feedback, it's up to you to dig in a little, asking for ways your boss thinks you might improve or for opportunities to take on more responsibilities than you've currently got. Seek criticism and coaching in your areas of deficit. Help your boss prepare for your annual review by compiling a list of your accomplishments, a self-assessment, and other information. Accept and appreciate criticism without defensiveness, and be grateful for opportunities to improve.

In some situations in professional life, the employee–boss relationship sours and doesn't appear easily fixable. When it's not going well, your boss holds the key to your short-term future in that he can release you at any time—a terrifying position to be in, in any economy. Some bosses might unconsciously marginalize their employees by not communicating or by giving desirable projects to and allying themselves with others. If you sense that something has shifted in your relationship with your boss or that communication is dropping off, take it as a sign to either sort things out or move on (see Lessons 49 and 50). Don't depart in an emotional flounce or with a dramatic exit, however. If you move on to another post, analyze how you might have better managed your boss—and then, when you're employed again, do things differently so it doesn't happen again.

EXERCISE 1

Think about a time when things didn't go well with your boss. How could you have managed the situation differently? What personal values or approaches were in conflict? What did you learn from that experience that you will carry forward?

EXERCISE 2

When a situation with your boss doesn't go as you had planned and you have lingering hurt or angry feelings, rather than send the unpleasantness to a compartment deep inside, take charge of it. How will you address the situation in a follow-up conversation without sounding defensive or apologizing for your viewpoint? Write about this experience in your journal.

RESOURCE

Gabarro, J. J., and J. Kotter. 2008. *Managing Your Boss.* Cambridge, MA: Harvard Business Review Press.

Engage and Align
with Physicians

No one argues with doing what is right for patients. The
art of servant leadership is finding ways to make it easier
for members of the healthcare team to operationalize.
The best leaders respond with "How?" not "No."

—*Jonathon D. Truwit, MD, MBA,*
enterprise chief medical officer and senior administrative dean,
Froedtert & the Medical College of Wisconsin, Milwaukee

PHYSICIAN–ADMINISTRATOR RELATIONSHIPS are often
cast as adversarial, even diametrically opposed. But why? Perhaps
strong professional boundaries, confusing payment structures, different foci, unaligned processes, and practice incentives cause the
divide.

However, the two groups are basically in sync. The physician
wants the best possible care for her patients. And although administrators are necessarily more wedded to the organization's bottom
line, they want exactly the same thing. So acknowledging at the
outset that their goals align is a positive place to begin.

How well you work with physicians is a major predictor of how
successful you'll be as a healthcare executive. Many administrators
who are successful at forging strong, honest, and respectful relationships with physicians are granted oversight of their organization's

hiring decisions because they've got a good track record of developing close personal and professional bonds.

When you engage and align yourself with physicians, you establish partnerships that make for the best patient care possible. So how do you do that?

- **Understand what physicians want.** Administrators should view problems from the physicians' vantage as well as their own and come up with solutions that give a nod to both sides. If you don't have a sense of what physicians want, ask. Be clear about what's at stake, and listen. Make sure that decisions aren't of the winner-take-all variety. Compromise so that both sides get something they want and no one feels they got the short end of the stick.

- **Build relationships.** Get to know your physicians. Ask them to describe the problems they face, and then help them find routes to meaningful and permanent solutions. Be the first to offer support for an issue, and grant favors that are within your power, big and small. Be a servant leader—someone who makes it easier for doctors to do their job. And be humble about it. Your ethic and efforts will be valued, remembered, and likely returned in kind.

- **Stand tall in your own skin while still maintaining humility.** Don't be fearful, intimidated, or starstruck by physicians' knowledge, power, or multiple academic degrees; they are human beings with pasts, wishes, fears, and goals just like you. Dealing comfortably with smart, successful physicians is crucial for your career as a healthcare executive. Remember, their role is different but not necessarily more important. So be confident in your dealings with physicians. Like anyone, physicians can smell intimidation and may use it to their advantage—or as an excuse not to take you seriously.

- **Do what you say you will do.** Doctors and administrators often work in different time zones when it comes to decision making. Physicians need information for the diagnosis and treatment of their patients and often make decisions on the spot with the data they have. Thus, a physician may make numerous decisions about multiple patients in the same 30-minute visit to a patient floor. Administrators, on the other hand, need to get input and buy-in from others and must spend time investigating problems and researching apt solutions before solidifying their decision. For example, an administrator may spend many months working on next year's budget. So remember doctors' time constraints, and if you say you will get back to them, do it—or else you'll lose credibility. Be as prompt as possible.

- **Be flexible and accommodating.** It's the nature of the beast: Physicians have chaotic, intensely busy days with back-to-back patients, and they often have trouble making it to your office on time—or even during the business day. Therefore, go where they are: Be available when they have some downtime between surgeries, meet them in the doctors' lounge, or stop by their office after their last patient of the day. Don't make a big deal about bending over backwards—simply anticipate that you'll need to accommodate them.

- **Speak respectfully to and about your physician colleagues.** Never complain about physicians to anyone, and never engage in conflict with a doctor in public. Your physician colleagues must feel that you are trustworthy and respectful and that you value them, their role, and their work. Expect the same of them.

- **Do your best to involve physicians in decisions and plans.** Often, physicians are brought in at the last minute to approve a new piece of equipment, lend support for a new program, or confirm a forthcoming policy change. They're busy, of course. But although they may not be able to attend meetings or thoroughly read the material you send to them, they do likely want to be involved in decisions that affect their work. Figure out how to include them in your organization's processes and decisions early on so that it's not a fire drill for support when decision time comes.

- **Identify and ally yourself with informal physician leaders.** A few physicians have powerful medical and social influence—as well as the intense respect of their colleagues. Though it may not be readily apparent early on in your tenure who these individuals are—particularly given that many thought leaders aren't necessarily the most vocal—do your best to seek them out and establish rapport and trust with them.

- **Be consistent in your messages.** Sometimes a healthcare manager says no to a physician, and the physician then appeals to the CEO, who reverses the decision. This kind of sequence not only disempowers the original manager; it also undermines respect for other managers and sends the message to physicians that the administrative team lacks consensus. Before saying yes or no to a physician's request, limit your authority by saying that you need to check with others who know more about the issue than you.

- **Reward and recognize.** Physicians offer a great deal of themselves, their time, and their energy to patient care and service for your organization, and although they enjoy a certain degree of glory, everyone likes to be thanked. You can recognize physicians' commitment in both financial and nonmonetary ways, but remember that a financial reward must come in tandem with a meaningful thank-you (especially given that a $1,000 bonus on its own might seem a little anemic to a physician making six figures). Sending a handwritten thank-you note is an effective and memorable way to personalize your appreciation for a physician.

Early in your career, get in the habit of learning as much as you can about your physician colleagues, both personally and professionally. Learn the language of and be interested in medicine as best you can. Read about health issues, and express genuine curiosity about what the doctors you work with do and face. Ask if you can spend time observing them in the operating room or accompanying them on rounds.

Remember, you're both there for the same reason: to do what is best for the patient.

EXERCISE 1

Spend time with physicians. Learn what they do. Ask to observe them in the operating room or on rounds.

EXERCISE 2

Learn the clinical language of physicians. Take a medical terminology course. Practice reading the operating room schedule and looking up words you don't know.

RESOURCES

Bujak, J. S. 2008. *Inside the Physician Mind: Finding Common Ground with Doctors.* Chicago: Health Administration Press.

Fields, R. 2011. "7 Reasons Hospitals Struggle to Align with Physicians." *Becker's Hospital Review.* Published July 29. www .beckershospitalreview.com/hospital-physician-relationships /7-reasons-hospitals-struggle-to-align-with-physicians.html.

Build and Support Strong Teams

Nurses learn very little about doctors in nursing school,
and doctors learn very little about nurses in medical school.
In the hospital we come together from this position of
relative ignorance, expected to work closely, often on
matters of life and death. Why anyone thinks that's a good
strategy for effective healthcare is a mystery to me.

—*Theresa Brown, PhD, BSN, RN,*
clinical nurse, New York Times opinion columnist,
and author of Critical Care: A New Nurse Faces Death,
Life and Everything in Between

IMAGINE FOR A moment all the special knowledge it takes to
perform open-heart surgery, a procedure in which many professionals work together in an elaborately choreographed production
to ensure a patient receives the best, most thorough care possible.
We take it for granted that strong, communicative, interdisciplinary teams just happen—but the truth is that collaborative teams
are usually carefully cultivated.

Twenty-first century healthcare delivery is a team business. We
may rotate in and out of teams several times every day, working
across professional lines, adroitly moving in and out of physical
environments, varying our roles, and collaborating with a range of
experts. That is the nature of healthcare and the nature of seamless
and coordinated delivery.

The airline industry has long understood the criticality of collaborative care and spends a great deal of time and energy training its employees to be effective team members. Healthcare is increasingly coming to understand that it, too, must follow the airlines' example, investing in interprofessional training so that, ultimately, the patient, clinician, and organization all benefit.

Whether from coursework or ancillary reading, most healthcare managers are familiar with the concept of high-reliability organizations. These organizations—in industries such as healthcare and aviation—must rely on teamwork for synchronicity, anticipation, real-time adjustments, deference to expertise, and knowing what to do quickly when things go awry. If you are that patient on the operating room table or that passenger 30,000 feet in the air during a crisis, you hope there is a team that knows what to do (and has practiced its moves) should an emergency take place. The key point here is that a high-performing team can make all the difference in the world in terms of outcome.

Members of high-performing teams must have a great degree of trust and belief in one another. Airline crews are frequently different for each flight, and they may not know their peers intimately, but they share a job and goal—the safety of passengers—that informs their every move. As you progress in your career, the way you champion teamwork will be crucial to your—and your organization's—success.

To develop and support strong interprofessional teams, you should do the following:

- **Dedicate resources to initial and ongoing teamwork training.** Teams don't just materialize out of thin air. They're nurtured, trained in what makes a good team, and taught the technical skills required to act nimbly when unanticipated events occur.
- **Get the right people on the team.** Mix it up. If yours is a performance improvement team, for example, add a financial analyst to solve problems related to patient

throughput. Varied perspectives add richness and will fortify a more robust response.

- **Encourage interprofessional education and collaboration.** Clinical improvement teams need to be supported with training, resources, and tools. If your nurses and therapists are not involved in patient rounds every day, they must begin immediately. If you work in a teaching hospital with medical and nursing students, champion education across professional boundaries. If your organization is not an academic medical center, you can still get nurses and doctors together for continuing education. Talk it up, offer readings and resources, and let your platform be that working together well really matters.

- **Train for leadership and followership.** Your role on the team may change as needs and members shift. One day you may be the leader and the next a follower—and that's OK. Learn that your role as a leader may sometimes be to follow in lockstep with your colleagues behind someone else's instruction. Too many leaders can be a recipe for disaster and inefficiency.

- **Have checklists, but don't be a slave to them.** Such tools are good for quality purposes and help ensure that the steps taken are evidence based to yield positive outcomes. However, checklists followed mindlessly may lead to problems. So pay attention to the qualitative aspects of the tasks at hand. If the patient or problem doesn't fit neatly into a checklist, then use your professional judgment— and the expertise of your team—to make an exception and find a better pathway.

- **Fix systems and processes to support teams.** If nurses are not rounding with doctors every day because each patient has a different doctor and doctors complain that they have to visit a dozen different units to see their patients, fix the issue. Your job as a manager is to do the behind-the-scenes organizational and administrative work so that the caregiving teams can concentrate on patient care, not worry about logistical details.

- **Make sure each team member understands—and respects—the other team members' jobs.** Synchronicity can occur only when team members are both competent and in firm agreement that their team is most effective working as a whole rather than individually.
- **Offer rewards.** High-performing teams may receive nonfinancial rewards from the positive outcomes of their interventions—the satisfaction of doing a job well, for example. As a manager, however, know your outstanding teams and reward them both monetarily and through recognition and praise. You don't need to wait until an extraordinary event takes place to do so; recognize teams that work together well every day, and acknowledge that their work is critical and prevents medical errors.

Excellent teamwork can be also described as group or organizational mindfulness because teams must be in the moment, work together, and anticipate a full range of next steps. They must pick up on subtle cues, tap their vast reservoirs of nursing and medical knowledge, and, above all, communicate with one another.

But interprofessional agility isn't experienced only in the hospital; it can also take place in the boardroom. Notice people's body language and tone of voice, and be prepared to take your proposal or discussion in a different direction, if necessary, to ensure you're working together with your colleagues in the best manner possible.

Teams truly are at the center of providing care to patients and their families, and it is incumbent on you, the manager, to champion effective teamwork, provide resources to train teams, and recognize and reward their contributions. Working on a team that works together for the good of the patient is the greatest feeling in healthcare. We hope that you have this experience!

EXERCISE 1

Ask one of your heart surgeons if you can shadow his team to learn more about effective teamwork.

EXERCISE 2

Attend a teamwork training session, and put what you learn into practice. Many business schools offer such seminars and skills training workshops.

RESOURCES

Mosser, G., and J. W. Begun. 2013. *Understanding Teamwork in Health Care.* New York: McGraw-Hill Education.

Weiss, D., F. Tilin, and M. J. Morgan. 2013. *The Interprofessional Health Care Team: Leadership and Development.* Burlington, MA: Jones & Bartlett Learning.

Find and Fix Problems

When solving problems, first identify the problem, get the facts, and then craft an appropriate, targeted solution. Often, the perception of a problem causes people to panic and launch "solutions" that are unrelated to the real problem. Respond quickly, but respond with a plan that remedies the right issues.

—K. Roger Johnson Jr.,
founding partner, Ivy Ventures,
Richmond, Virginia

THE MOST IMPORTANT skill of *any* manager's job in *any* field—healthcare included—is the ability to recognize, define, and figure out solutions to problems. Effective problem solvers will always have career opportunities because of their ability to break down issues and chart a path toward positive change.

The best way to learn to deal with issues is by working out *real* problems in *real* organizations, big and small. But you have to start somewhere. So if you're fresh out of school and in the early days of your very first job, seek assignments that allow you to tackle issues and gain problem-solving experience. Volunteer, if necessary. Don't be afraid of challenges, because you truly will learn by doing.

If you can, find out whether your company takes a formal or informal approach to solving problems. Many organizations now use frameworks such as Lean and Six Sigma, and if your company is among these organizations, become an expert in these techniques. Some places offer problem-solving training in-house or at local universities or other training facilities to hone their administrators' skills in analyzing issues. Certifications might even be useful—the University of Michigan, for example, offers courses that lead to healthcare Lean and Six Sigma certification—so if a formal path is available to boost your problem-solving skills, make a case to attend.

Every problem is different, of course, but a systematic approach is prudent no matter what the issue is:

- **Recognize and define the problem.** This first step is often the most difficult. All too often, executives "solve" what they thought was the real problem only to discover that the problem persists after a great deal of attention, effort, and money has been spent on it. For example, a hospital that is suffering from declines in outpatient volume might think the root of the problem has to do with their lack of branding. But even after a multimillion-dollar marketing and branding campaign, the problem of declining volumes might remain because the *real* problem was related to quality. As you define the problem, be honest—not hopeful. This is not the time to initiate an off-target pet project.

- **Focus on understanding the issue.** Hold frank discussions with both internal and external stakeholders to fully understand the parameters of the problem. Note every facet of the organization that the problem touches. Once the problem has been isolated, the solution will likely be straightforward.

- **Gather the *real* facts.** Everyone in the organization may assert that admissions are dropping because Dr. Jones is angry at the administrator or because Dr. Smith has a bad attitude and patients and staff find him difficult to work with. Don't let yourself be distracted by false, superficial claims. Problems usually have basic, simple, obvious sources, and hurt feelings and office politics generally aren't at the root. Use Occam's razor—the principle that, of all possible solutions, the one involving the fewest assumptions is usually correct—to define what ails your organization. The simplest, most obvious, and most straightforward solution is likely the truest and the best answer.

- **Analyze the problem from all angles.** How much does the problem cost? What are the potential benefits if it's solved? If feasible, capture the problem in numbers and narrative. Simplify it to its very essence. Remember that, as the problem-solver-in-chief, you are responsible for presenting your findings succinctly. Keep your bullet points clear, clean, and concise. Develop a 60- to 90-second "elevator speech" about it for on-the-fly conversations and questions. Supporting information, research, and analysis should be close at hand for easy reference.

- **Talk it through, and listen well.** If you take time to listen to as many people as you can about a problem and how to solve it, a solution will crystallize. Know how to listen. Your chance to speak will come when you make a decision about a fix.

- **Share possible solutions with your constituents.** Engage in healthy discussions about solutions and their impacts. What are the pros and cons of each? As particular pathways out of the problem present themselves, get a sense of how people feel about each one. Consensus about a direction is key.

- **Decide on a course of action.** Do your best to ensure colleagues and stakeholders concur about what route to take. Expend extra effort to make sure practitioners will embrace and follow changes. Be sure to involve clinicians in defining the problem and its solution.

- **Remain involved.** Continue to monitor the issue carefully, and chart the path to change until you see that progress has been achieved. Once a positive, preselected metric is reached and the problem appears to subside, assign follow-up efforts to a trusted colleague. Meet with that colleague regularly to make sure progress in the right direction is being made.

- **Establish a metric for the successful solution of the project.** Let employees know when the measure is reached, and thank everyone for their support. Should the measure not be reached in the designated time frame, reconvene and chart a modified plan to accomplish the established metric of success.

Problem-solving skills are honed with practice, and your thoughtful study and analysis of problems will earn you praise and regard—and give you stamina to solve the next set of issues that crop up. Remember that the issues you successfully address will not only help your organization's bottom line—they will also add another notch to your professional experience belt and prepare you for future roles.

EXERCISE 1

Keep a journal of the problems you have solved. What skills did you use? What worked, and what didn't? Routinely study your journal to look for patterns that will help you hone your skills. Seek input and counsel from your supervisor.

EXERCISE 2

Find out as much as you can about the problem-solving method that your organization uses. Study the problem-solving techniques of an organization you admire.

EXERCISE 3

Make a list of all of your projects. Is it clear who is responsible for each project's completion? Does the person responsible for completing each project have a level of authority that is commensurate with the project's scope of responsibility?

RESOURCES

Graban, M. 2012. *Lean Hospitals: Improving Quality, Patient Safety, and Employee Engagement*, second edition. Boca Raton, FL: CRC Press.

Johns Hopkins Medicine Center for Innovation in Quality Patient Care. 2014. "What Is Lean Sigma?" Accessed November 11. www.hopkinsmedicine.org/innovation _quality_patient_care/areas_expertise/lean_sigma/about/.

University of Michigan College of Engineering. 2014. "Lean Healthcare: Combining World-Class Lean Healthcare Training Expertise with Hands-On Experience." Professional program. Accessed November 11. http://isd.engin.umich.edu /professional-programs/lean-healthcare/index.htm.

Be Visible by Rounding

How can executives understand the needs of patients, physicians, and nurses without interacting with them on a daily basis? When I walk through the hospital, it is a great opportunity to gather information and build trust by listening and responding to concerns. Rounding takes me beyond the paper dashboard so I can get a true pulse on the health of the organization. It's been the key to my success as CEO.

—*Mike Sherrod,*
CEO, Coliseum Northside Hospital,
Macon, Georgia

SUCCESSFUL EXECUTIVES KNOW that being visible in their organization is critical. The best healthcare leaders get out of their offices, roam the halls and unit corridors, chat with employees, and discover what's going on outside the confines of their usual areas of responsibility. They're engaging, approachable, and curious, and they listen well. Often, they're beloved simply because they're seen, they care enough to take in the work of others, and they're not uncomfortable when outside the hallowed walls of the executive suite communicating with people who aren't wearing suits.

You can easily fill your calendar each day with meetings and calls and get caught up with daily activities that make you lose sight of *who* makes the organization hum and *how*. If you have an assistant, make sure you control your calendar and personally approve its entries. Be selective with your time so that you're able to fit in 30 to 60 minutes of rounds at least several times each week. Visibility is truly a key to executive success.

Rounding brings a bounty of benefits. It can be a great way to get buy-in from colleagues, to gather information about your company's culture, and to spread word about your ideas and initiatives. Executives who round show that they understand and appreciate their employees' hard work and dedication, and people will follow leaders who take time to talk, listen, and explain their decisions. Although employees may not always agree with the leaders' decisions, they will respect their forthcoming attitude because they're there, in the trenches, taking the time to listen and learn.

The key to successful rounding is to do it regularly but not predictably. Make your approach at different times of day. Follow different routes, taking different corridors and elevators. Don't forget to visit places that aren't on the way to anywhere—the loading dock, for example, or the mailroom or cafeteria. Round on weekend and holiday shifts, if you can. Offer special praise to those who work during off-hours. Ask people what they're working on and how it's going. And don't rush it. You'll be appreciated for your presence—and you'll have the opportunity to appreciate others.

Other aspects to successful rounding include the following:

- Call people by name, and introduce yourself to those you don't know.
- Express admiration for and curiosity about others' work and work strategies—and remember to offer your thanks.
- Smile, be approachable, and be ready to talk to anyone who wishes to speak to you.
- If you see something exceptional or someone going beyond the call of duty, offer praise—and take note of it. Those who do good when no one's looking may be great people to tap for an award, promotion, or raise.

- If appropriate, and time permitting, use your rounds to ask physicians, employees, and patients their opinion about any issues on your mind or theirs.
- Be respectful of the environment you're in. For example, if you're rounding in the intensive care unit or the emergency department, be sensitive in particular to the patients there as well as the tempo and stress levels of those caring for them.
- Remember to jot down notes so that, if you make a promise to do something, you'll remember to follow up. People always remember those who do what they say they're going to do because such behavior is rather rare. *Be that rare leader.*

A guiding principle for rounding—and for most of your interactions, save the most difficult ones—is the Golden Rule: Treat people the way you would like to be treated. Understand and believe that every contribution is important to your organization's proper and successful function. If someone is cleaning bathrooms, catch them with a smile, a handshake, and an honest, nonpatronizing compliment: "Your work is critical to our success and patient satisfaction. When I see the hospital looking good, I feel great—and so do our patients!"

Rounding can also provide an opportunity to observe and curb lackluster or noncompliant behaviors. Take note of poor performance, and offer a private reminder to those exhibiting noncompliant behavior right then and there. If you see something out of order, communicate with the appropriate department leader and give them a chance to correct it. Be on the lookout for opportunities to improve the work environment and make the area safer for patients. Though you're not out to catch anyone acting poorly, take note of underperformers and weed them out, if need be. If you observe a situation that threatens the safety of patients or staff, you must take immediate corrective action.

Visiting all of the areas you're responsible for—and making appearances in areas where you're not in charge but that are integral to the organization's health—is one of the best ways to gather information and be an effective leader. Rounding truly represents the very best time you will spend each day.

EXERCISE 1

Do different things as you round each day, keeping some sort of numerical goal in mind. For example, one morning your goal might be to speak with five staff nurses. The next day, you could aim to speak with three physicians or two housekeepers. One day, try to visit three units that you haven't visited in a month.

EXERCISE 2

Make a point of meeting new people each day, and remember their names.

RESOURCES

Cleary, P. R., and J. S. Lindsey. 2013. "Navy Captain's Advice to the C-Suite: 5 Simple Leadership Tenets That Will Make Your Hospital Shine." *Becker's Hospital Review.* Published July 18. www.beckershospitalreview.com/white-papers/navy -captain-s-advice-to-the-c-suite-5-simple-leadership-tenets -that-will-make-your-hospital-shine.html.

Lindsey, J. S., and B. Corkran. 2012. "4 Keys to Effective Administrative Rounding." *Becker's Hospital Review.* Published May 22. www.beckershospitalreview.com /hospital-management-administration/4-keys-to-effective -administrative-rounding.html.

Reward and Celebrate

I truly believe that "thank you" and "I appreciate you" are magic words. They change relationships and inspire others in ways that no other words, data, or formal incentive programs can. The hardest part, I've found, is getting started and finding your own voice so that your recognition is authentic.

I write a lot of thank-you notes—always handwritten and personal. Over the years, people have told me how much these notes have meant to them. Right now, my desk has thank-you notes from students, colleagues, and alumni. When I am feeling frustrated or challenged, I grab one of these and reread it. I am instantly reminded why I do the work that I do. One of my first tips for graduate students is to buy a box of thank-you notes and have them on hand, because you never know when you might want to share some "magic words."

—*Christy Harris Lemak, PhD, FACHE,*
professor and chair, Department of Health Services Administration,
University of Alabama at Birmingham

IN THE LEADERSHIP courses we have taught for many years in both traditional and executive formats, our students consistently report that they don't feel adept at offering rewards and celebrating their employees. Of course, everyone among us appreciates being rewarded for what we do—and what we do well—so how can we be better at responding to this very basic human need to belong, to be cherished, and to be respected for our contributions? Why is doling out this kind of appreciation so difficult?

Although we usually blame a perceived lack of time to properly offer thanks and praise to our colleagues, the fact is that rewards and recognition feel tricky because you have to know the people with whom you work and whether they like public or individual recognition. Rewarding teams, work units, and departments feels safer and easier because you don't risk embarrassing or offending someone on the receiving end of praise. But just because it's hard or has the potential for making people feel awkward doesn't mean it should be skipped.

If you are mindful of praising yourself, the task of rewarding others may come a bit more easily. Many of us need to take time to soak in the feeling of accomplishment after finishing a big task, before darting off to what's next. As you experience your own successes, be mindful of what has occurred, and mark the occasion. Some colleagues celebrate accomplishments with a ceremony or ritual, such as a fancy dinner out after coming in under budget, successfully opening a new service, publishing a journal article or book, or completing a successful accreditation site visit. Such rituals offer us time to reflect on what worked and what didn't and to set new goals for working together in the future.

Similar celebrations of goals, important dates such as national nurses' or doctors' days, or the anniversary of your organization's founding are all moments to mark what has been done, offer reverence to a skill set, or recognize why those around you are special. And although having too many parties may be unwise (because moving from party to party can make you seem unsocial), simply acknowledging the need to reward and recognize is a great place to begin.

Here are some additional tips:

- **Be thoughtful.** If someone goes the extra mile for you or your organization, thank them. Keep a stack of $5 gift cards to coffee or sandwich shops in your desk and enclose one with a thank-you note. Send flowers to someone who starts a new job. When a major initiative is successfully completed (e.g., an accreditation site visit) or a major goal is achieved, host a lunch for the key organizers to let them know you've noticed them and their work.

- **Handwrite notes.** Although e-mail often does the job, it doesn't pack the same punch as a handwritten note. And although different generations may prefer different communication methods, a handwritten note is universally pleasing—and increasingly out of the ordinary.

- **Catch people doing good.** When you see people going beyond what is expected for a patient or hear about a situation that reflects your organization's mission and values, recognize it personally and praise it publicly. Remember people's past contributions, too: "It was Bill's idea to try this in the pediatric intensive care unit—and look at the results!"

- **Keep your praise specific.** "Good job!" refrains lose their meaning if they're not tied to something specific. You might say, "I saw how you handled that difficult customer over the chaos of ringing phones, and how you kept your cool as you walked her to where she needed to go. I'm impressed—and grateful." Name specific behaviors, such as compassion, patience, and handling specific customer needs with a smile. Mention the strength to the person's supervisor, if that's not you. If your organization has formal opportunities to nominate someone for doing good, take advantage of them. Be a serial nominator for these kinds of awards, offering praise whenever you see it's deserved.

- **Tune in to your network.** Don't remember to be kind to your network contacts only when you need them; offer praise routinely when you hear about their professional accomplishments. When someone gets a new job or achieves the FACHE credential, send them a note of congratulations. You can't go wrong with this kind of praise and connection, and you never know when or why such gestures will be recalled.

- **Remember birthdays.** Doing so is far easier than you might imagine. Add your colleagues' birthdays to your e-mail calendar such that you are reminded a day or two in advance. Keep a stash of birthday cards in your desk drawer, or plan to call, e-mail, or salute them in the hallway. As grownups, we don't put the same huge investment in birthdays as we did when we were kids, but it's fabulous when someone remembers ours.

- **Take team pictures, and post them.** Reinforce how people in your organization are connected by a common purpose—and show they can have fun, too.

- **Be good at names.** Remembering names is hard for many. But once you start being mindful about it, remembering names—even hundreds if not thousands of them— will come more easily to you. Just use a mnemonic or alliteration to connect the person's name to something that you will remember. Becky, for instance, is in charge of the building.

- **Reinforce outstanding performance in your messaging.** When you communicate to others, whatever the format, include positive stories about your associates—examples of excellent teamwork, devotion to and connection with the organization's mission, someone you "caught" doing a good deed, or an anecdote about your organization's founder that humanizes, informs, and brings him closer to the mission and tone of the place.

- **Be inclusive.** Keep in mind that in healthcare, much of your workforce is there 24/7. Evening, night, and weekend staff often don't get noticed the same way that the 9-to-5ers do. Show up with pizza on the night shift, or make rounds on a holiday. Word will travel like wildfire through the organization that you really care—and that you're willing to make a real effort.

- **Exhibit compassion.** When things don't go well and your people are anxious, remember that they need attention, too. Listen, console, and affirm. Don't focus all your attention on the superstars or reserve praise and connection only for when things are going swimmingly. Remember that many of your people are plugging away, day after day, doing their jobs without fanfare or reward—and that their jobs are critical to your organization's smooth operation. Find a way to thank everyone, acknowledge what they do, and recognize how they contribute.

All of us engaged in healthcare have a calling to serve people. We all want to know that our work is bigger than us and that it truly makes a difference. As leaders, we must practice rewarding others and celebrating not only what they do in work but who they are as people. In our profession, it *all* matters.

EXERCISE 1

Keep a list of things to celebrate and people to thank. Keep a stack of thank-you notes and birthday cards, and use them.

EXERCISE 2

Discuss celebrations with your staff, and develop a positive culture of celebration that is focused on helping people.

RESOURCE

Kouzes, J. M., and B. Z. Posner. 2003. *Encouraging the Heart: A Leader's Guide to Rewarding and Recognizing Others.* San Francisco: Jossey-Bass.

Innovate

Innovation requires perspiration as well as inspiration.
There is an art and science to evaluating whether an
innovation is viable and how to turn an innovation
into a successful do good–do well venture.

—*Regina E. Herzlinger, PhD,*
professor, Harvard Business School,
Cambridge, Massachusetts

INNOVATION IN HEALTHCARE reveals new and better ways to solve existing problems and overhaul complicated systems. Innovative leaders not only tackle issues in outside-the-box ways; they also get things done—and get noticed. Although the "secret sauce" of innovation is made from a multifaceted recipe of perspective, planning, and approach, innovation itself is nothing more than taking existing ideas, technology, and procedures and reshaping them to produce a superior product, a better procedure, or novel, top-notch services. Innovators take old ideas and do them in new and better ways.

Of course, they have to be the right ideas—ones that are aligned with organizational goals and that have the potential to be malleable, reproducible, and entrepreneurial. And innovation usually involves change, sometimes of the 180-degree variety. But of course, such change is necessary for organizations that aim to get better, stronger, and more tuned in to the marketplace so that they can transform their relevancy to current and future environments. Particularly in a field as dynamic and ever-changing as healthcare, we can't simply do everything as we've always done it and expect to be at the top of our game. Change, in this profession in particular, is essential.

Apple Inc. is often cited as one of the most innovative companies of the last two decades. Led by visionary Steve Jobs, Apple not only found an interface that worked well for customers, but its platforms and products also brought technology to consumers in a whole new way: brilliantly designed, accessible, and technologically friendly. Before Apple, technology had never involved beautiful design, but Apple turned that notion on its head by making products that engaged humans on a very human level, appealing to them in very human ways. And how it worked!

Like computers in the era before Apple, healthcare is a field that is sorely overdue for beautiful, thoughtful, creatively conceived ideas that truly serve the customer. As cumbersome as it has become, with layer upon layer of providers, laboratories, equipment, and countless billing offices, the industry has a host of parts that could be made better, more accessible, more user-friendly— and far more human. A scheduling system that allows patients to make appointments with their providers quickly and easily is one example of a system component that could be overhauled in an innovative fashion. Ways to deconstruct common medical procedures or to choose a primary care provider based on reviews are other components long in need of an overhaul. A billing system that enables patients to see and understand their costs for any given procedure up front, based on the insurance they have and the procedures they anticipate having done, is another area that could use attention. You might consider what issue in your organization ensnares and maddens the most customers, clinicians, and others—and then move in to begin your own innovation.

So how you can make things move better and faster? Here are a few questions to consider at the outset:

- Keeping your organization's current strengths in mind, what new products or services spring to mind that would not involve a huge investment in capital?
- What problems does your organization face, and how might you rethink how those problems are solved and addressed?
- What resources and individuals do you need to bring about the change you're eyeing?
- Who are your most forward-thinking colleagues, and can they help you determine innovative solutions to problems your organization faces?
- Are your target innovations in line with your organization's strategic goals and culture?
- Can you ally yourself with any external strategic partners and use your collective strengths to offer a new product or better service?
- Once your innovation is implemented, how and with whom will you need to communicate to ensure that it becomes the "new normal"? How will you measure whether it's working, and who is responsible for making it work?
- Is your innovation sustainable?

Robert Tucker's *Innovation Is Everybody's Business* offers seven ways to prepare for innovative opportunities:

1. **Consciously shift your perspective.** Think of problems as opportunities, and brainstorm ways to fix them.
2. **Think small.** Not every innovation has to be a massive overhaul. Fixing small things can make a difference, too—often greater than you'd imagine. Look for opportunities where you are, the proverbial "low-hanging fruit."

3. **Listen for "there's got to be a better way" mutterings.**
   For every annoyance, there is likely a simpler, more
   efficient, more elegant way to go.

4. **Pay attention to happy accidents.** Remember penicillin?
   An intended use for one product or service may wind
   up being useful in other ways. Serendipity also plays an
   important role, so pay attention to chance meetings and
   unexpected encounters that can add value.

5. **Examine customer problems that aren't being solved.**
   Healthcare has a lot of these—and has earned a reputation
   for overcomplicating procedures and policies that should
   be much simpler. Usually, the simplest solution is the
   best. Look for trends and issues that repeatedly crop up
   in patient satisfaction surveys (the food, the waste, the
   inexplicable billing) and aim to address big problems
   simply, creatively, and efficiently.

6. **Eliminate non-value-adding work.** What can we stop
   doing that isn't making a difference? And how can we
   spend the time gained on opportunities to solve problems
   creatively?

7. **Think big—but remember that problems of all sizes
   matter.** The innovator looks at things not as they are but as
   they could and should be. Have a vision, and don't be afraid
   to tackle an issue that seems mountain sized—yet don't
   ignore the one that's hill sized, either. All change matters—
   and making one thing that everyone faces in a healthcare
   system easier shows thought, bravery, and fortitude.

We stand at the precipice of true change in our profession, a
time when large healthcare organizations are looking at ways to
reduce waste, cut costs, and offer better, safer, higher-quality care
with a leaner, better educated, more customer-centered staff. And
whether we like it or not, change is coming hard and fast because,
for far too long, healthcare organizations have complacently

obfuscated and overcomplicated systems that shouldn't be so. By assuming a fearless posture and inquisitive mind as you determine ways to innovate and change your organization, you'll be leading a profession that must figure out what it will ultimately become—and how. Change is the only static in healthcare; that is for certain.

EXERCISE 1

As you build your network, seek to meet creative, idea-generating people. Ask colleagues in other organizations what issues they've tackled and how.

EXERCISE 2

Make a list of problems, and think of innovative ways to solve them by looking at case studies, speaking with colleagues in other organizations, and chatting with the peers you work with. What do you do well? What things that you do well might be expanded on? What things could you do better?

RESOURCES

Clark, B., and S. Lindsey. 2013. "5 Ways Innovation Can Save YourHospital." *Becker's Hospital Review.* Published September 16. www.beckershospitalreview.com/hospital -management-administration/5-ways-innovation-could-save -your-hospital.html.

Drucker, P. F. 1998. "The Discipline of Innovation." *Harvard Business Review* 76 (6): 149–57.

Herzlinger, R. E. 2014. "Innovating in Health Care—Framework." Harvard Business School Case No. 314-017. Boston: Harvard Business School Press.

Tucker, R. B. 2011. *Innovation Is Everybody's Business.* Hoboken, NJ: John Wiley & Sons.

Motivate and Engage
Individuals and Teams

Engaging and motivating teams requires equal parts humility
and curiosity. Leaders will only get the best ideas and
commitment to see them through by asking their team for
input and then considering their contributions. A principle of
Lean organizations is that frontline employees are engaged by
leaders to brainstorm and test solutions because they are so
intimately involved in the processes and know the opportunities.
This way, leaders will most likely achieve the desired results
while improving employee commitment to the effort.

*—F. Matthew Gitzinger, MHA,
director, Office of the Chief Medical Information Officer,
Vidant Health,
Greenville, North Carolina*

SUCCESS ISN'T JUST having employees with the right ingredients;
it often comes when motivation and engagement are channeled
from the top. Strong leaders know how to pick talented, dedicated, visionary employees and partners, foster a can-do approach,
and cultivate momentum by gently urging and nurturing the
wire frame of success into shape en masse. But in large organizations especially, success tends to be collective in spirit—not of the
go-it-alone variety. So if "good people beget success," as Dr.
Thomas Frist Sr., one of HCA's founders, asserts, it's also true that

people love to be empowered to have ownership in and be part of a winning team. And real leaders can cultivate just that.

Good leaders know how to motivate people to work toward common goals and to achieve positive, value-adding results—and organizations are always on the hunt for managers who can inspire these traits in people. Any successful motivator must begin by leading with energy, conviction, and passion—with that, the excitement rubs off on the team. The best leaders also inspire individuals to become engaged and committed to the organization and their jobs and to be willing to go that extra mile. If you're not able to motivate and engage your team to rally around the organization's goals, your results won't be of the highest possible quality.

The best leaders engage and empower people to recognize that the work they do is vital to the organization's mission, vision, and operation. They take an interest in individuals and help them feel vitally important, like a crucial part of the machinery that makes the place go. Employees, of course, like to know that their leader is united with them and appreciates how hard they're working. Once they understand a project and their role in it, if properly motivated and reinforced, they'll work hard to achieve the organization's mission. And the best leaders always offer their heartiest thanks and praise.

Though the following advice may seem commonsensical, many managers don't cultivate these habits—and they pay a price for it. As your career grows and you develop your own style of managing and leading, pay attention to these tips to nurture motivation and engagement among your troops:

- **Have a clear vision.** Repeatedly articulating the organization's mission, vision, and values is a way to micronize them for individuals and teams. Understand what needs to be done and what the team's role is in doing it. Get input from your staff and others before making important decisions, and enable your team to have a say in what's decided and what will be achieved.

- **Choose the right projects, and don't bite off more than you can chew.** "Management is doing things right; leadership is doing the right things," writes business guru Peter Drucker—a sentiment that underscores how critical working on the right projects for the right reasons is. Great leaders learn to focus at the levels that move their organization forward, knowing the difference between simple actions and actual results. If you breathlessly spin through your workday without achieving goals that speak to your mission or vision, you're spreading yourself too thin and being ineffective. Don't take on too much at once. Learn to focus, and select three to five goals at any given point. Doing so will lend focus to your team—and will ensure that they do what they set out to do thoughtfully, thoroughly, and well.

- **Dissect and delegate.** Figure out what's to be done and who will be responsible for each component part. Make assignments thoughtfully. Does the task fit the skills of the person who will be tackling it? Who are your most engaged workers? And does the person you're assigning to do the job have the authority, training, and tools needed to complete it?

- **Enable and fortify.** Give employees what they want and need. Don't assume they have all the skills or tools they need to get the job done—check in with them personally and find out.

- **Ask, don't tell.** Everyone prefers to be asked to complete a job rather than be told what to do. Ask for opinions, best routes, and the like to enable and engage your colleagues and cultivate their ownership in the process. And be teachable. Have *them* tell *you* what they perceive is best—and if you concur, let them determine major components of the route or action plan.

- **Say why it's important, and ask for input.** Paint a picture of the issue, giving whatever details you have. "Our goal," you might say, "is to improve flow into and out of the operating room so that our patients won't be kept waiting as long. What ideas do you have? What can we do here?" Although you may know the desired outcome, your team may offer a variety of routes toward it that you hadn't previously considered. They'll also have a vested interest if they are empowered to come up with ideas to accomplish results.

- **Coach for success—and say thank you.** Feedback is a powerful motivator. Don't wait for their annual review to sing your colleagues' praises. Offer feedback (positive or gently negative) right away and as often as possible. Schedule regular meetings for updates and coaching. Show you're interested and available. And always remember to say thank you, which is a huge reward in itself.

- **Be respectful, kind, fair, and trustworthy.** Create a supportive, healthy work environment. Respect confidences, and never get angry or send mixed messages. Don't embarrass employees in front of others. When problems arise, understand the context by examining all sides, and if the problem is yours to solve, make a decision. If you make a mistake, admit you were wrong and apologize. And never be afraid to laugh at yourself.

- **Care about people—not just their results.** Take the time to get to know your employees, and always return their phone calls and e-mails. Be visible, check in for quick conversations to assess their workloads and stress levels, and offer help and resources if needed. Celebrate birthdays, and know in a general sense what issues they face at home. Recognize, too, that no one is tip-top 100 percent of the time. An off day is just that—be sure to look beyond it, especially when you've got a solidly talented crew.

- **Check in.** Take your employees' pulse from time to time, and understand how they feel about their progress toward a particular goal and any issues they're facing. Assess your team for diminishing engagement, flagging motivation, or exhaustion before it begins to crimp their progress and ultimate success. Ask them what needs changing and what's not going well—they'll tell you what needs to be done. Don't be afraid to take their suggestions and make midcourse corrections or pivots.

No one is an island. Your ability to engage and motivate people is among the most critical facets of your leadership. Cultivating these skills purposefully and thoughtfully through education and experience will only sharpen your abilities as a fearless, intrepid, and inspiring leader. Treat others the way you want to be treated, work hard yourself, and expect great things of your phenomenal team—and success will surely come.

EXERCISE 1

Rate yourself on your ability to engage and motivate your team. Map out a recent project, noting what went right—and what didn't. What might have been done better? Do a 360-degree review to understand the perception of the project's effectiveness. Record these results in your journal.

EXERCISE 2

Volunteer for a project that offers you the opportunity to motivate and engage people.

RESOURCE

Nelson, B. 2012. *1501 Ways to Reward Employees.* New York: Workman Publishing Company.

Take Charge of Your Career

EARLY IN MY career, I (Steve) was offered a job managing a five-hospital region by a colleague at a conference. I respected and trusted the person who offered me the job, so I said yes. The move was a pivotal stepping-stone in my career—but not because it was a perfect fit.

On the job, I learned that I didn't like being away from my family or having to travel every week and that being one step removed from the action as a regional manager was not as much fun as running a hospital—which engages all my senses and facilities in real time, before my very eyes.

A couple of years later, I heard that the leader of a hospital close to home, Henrico Doctors' Hospital, had resigned. I was tired of traveling, I missed my wife and family, and I missed working directly in the hospital environment. When I expressed my interest in the Henrico job to colleagues, everyone told me that the job would be a step down, that I would be making a huge mistake going back to a single-hospital gig, and that I would regret the move. I knew, however, that I ultimately wanted to be the CEO of a full-service hospital—and my gut told me this job was the route to achieving that goal. I had prepared for the job with my MHA degree and my experience in military leadership, financial management, and hospital operations. And when I became the CEO at Henrico, it confirmed that this career decision was the best I'd ever made—but it wouldn't have been possible without the heartaches I experienced and the knowledge I acquired from the jobs that came before.

Though the first six months of the CEO job were tough and riddled with doubt, things started to fall into place, and it became my dream job. I found an immense partner and mentor in Dr. Edward Martirosian, president of the hospital's board of directors, and together we worked to improve care in very real ways for patients at Henrico.

My point is that part of gleaning what you want is often based on experiencing what you don't want. I've found myself in bad situations from time to time—including one at a start-up healthcare company with a partner who had wholly different approaches to cost and quality than I did, a job in which I definitely stayed too long—but I always knew that each experience informed and enriched the next. When one door closes, another opens, and at every stop new lessons are learned, connections are made, and clarity is realized.

Such is the case for Ken, too. He once accepted a position as vice president of operations and then was told that either he or a colleague of the same rank would be named chief operating officer. The near-impossible competition and ill feelings that ensued were neither good for the organization nor for the people involved. Within two years Ken and his colleague had both moved on, still harboring uncomfortable feelings. A decade later they reconnected in an academic capacity. Health administration, Ken learned, is an intimate community—so never burn bridges.

Another lesson? Embrace serendipity. Ken came to health administration as a result of a series of school closings, forced transfers, and hallway conversations. Choosing nursing, then pivoting toward medicine, and then ultimately studying healthcare administration allowed him to sample each trajectory—and each, in turn, informed the way he worked with and understood clinicians, academics, and administrators. And he's never looked back.

One final story: I recall a former star student of ours who, after completing his master's, rapidly moved through the early phases of his career to become a hospital assistant administrator. But the job made him miserable, and he ultimately realized that he wasn't using his gifts. He'd always wanted to work with children and eventually became an elementary schoolteacher—and today he is a happy, well-adjusted associate principal. Sometimes we have to spend a lot of time, energy, and resources following one direction to find the correct path. We just need to be open to opportunities and not feel there are points in life where it's just "too late in the game."

Now that you've learned what it takes to manage yourself and your job—and perhaps had a few successes under your belt—you can begin to think about how to position yourself to take charge of your career.

Note that we've transitioned our language from the concept of "management" in the titles of the first two sections to "take charge" in this section. The idea is that you really can't take charge of your direction without first mastering yourself and your job. Once you've tackled the lessons in Sections I and II, where will you make your career take *you*?

—Steve Lindsey

Take Ownership of Your Career

When I advise young healthcare professionals, I remind
them to start with a vision based on their strengths. I tell
them to assess what they do well, as well as where they
need development, and then to compare their assets to
competencies that are strongly desirable in the field. Those
who demonstrate sound critical thinking and analytical skills
early on in their careers are the same ones who advance.

—*Jeff Dorsey, retired president and CEO,*
HCA Continental Division,
Denver, Colorado

YOU ALONE ARE responsible for managing your career. Although
your spouse, mentor, sponsor, coach, or boss may be invested and
interested in your success, it's solely up to you to determine the
particulars of your trajectory. *You* are the only one who can make
your professional dreams come true.

Develop a solid and honest understanding of yourself. Identify your gifts and your passions, and then set a course and create
career goals. Write out a professional development plan (or PDP;
see Lesson 41) for achieving those goals. Remember that this plan
is a fluid document and that all such plans must be flexible and
open to serendipity. Remember, too, that some of the jobs you will
hold over the course of your career probably have not even been
invented yet.

Focus your energy on solving problems and adding value to the company where you work. Don't waste energy blaming the environment, the economy, or others for what's wrong. Difficult issues and people will always exist, and your job is to solve those that are in your scope and to let go of others that are beyond your professional control. You will find that with intensity of purpose and focus, you can accomplish a great deal.

Here are some ideas to help you become the captain of your career ship:

- **Have a clear idea of what you want to do and what you're good at.** Do you want to be a hospital CEO or chief financial officer, or would you prefer to manage the human resource functions of a hospital? Are you interested in serving vulnerable populations? Are you attracted to academic medical centers, or do for-profit institutions excite you more? Consider geography, your desired salary, and the size and scope of the sort of institution you'd like to work in as well as your family's needs on the home front. Don't pursue opportunities or ideas that are clearly pipe dreams or so unrealistic that they're untenable. Be dreamy—but be grounded, too.
- **Write and maintain a PDP.** Be sure to review and update it at least every year.
- **Focus on doing exceptional work in your current job.** The best way to head toward a new, better job is to do your very best work in your current one. Employers seek executives with a proven track record of meaningful accomplishments. Find problems in your current gig, and solve them thoughtfully and competently.
- **Emphasize personal growth.** Learn new skills, expand your strengths, and stretch your limits. Your PDP will help you identify what to work on. Seek assignments that will challenge you.

- **Look beyond the confines of your job.** Young professionals often find themselves in positions with a very narrow focus. Broaden your horizon by volunteering for projects that expose you to larger issues in your organization. For example, you might volunteer to assess a community need and develop recommendations—and ultimately programs—to address that need. Along the way, you will probably meet people whom you can add to your professional network.

- **Seek out effective mentors.** "Ms. Smith," you might say, "I admire the way you work with the medical staff. Would you share with me some of the tactics you use?" Keep in mind that as a mentee, *you're* responsible for doing the most work. Some early careerists mistakenly think that they can just sit back and wait for their mentor to call them with advice. In point of fact, the mentee is the one who must pursue opportunities through the mentor— never forgetting to be unfailingly polite and grateful. Ask your mentor questions such as the following:

  - What's the next logical step up on the career ladder from my current job?
  - Do I have the education and experience required for that next step? If not, what degree, certification, or experience do I need to qualify?
  - Whom should I meet to begin the path toward my ideal job?

As you consider what's next, accept that if you're no longer learning and growing in your current position (even if you're still contributing), it is likely time to move on. It's *your* career and *your* life, and *you* should be the one who decides when and where to move on. Be the best captain you can be.

EXERCISE 1

Join the American College of Healthcare Executives (ACHE), and use the ACHE Career Management Network (a group of ACHE members who have volunteered to provide information and advice about career transitions in healthcare management). Even if you're not actively hunting for a new job, explore job opportunities online to keep apprised of what's currently available. Discuss the opportunities with close colleagues and with those in your network to get a sense of the positions' requirements (e.g., education, certifications, type and duration of previous work experience).

EXERCISE 2

Be realistic about what you're good at. Undergo a 360-degree evaluation to identify areas in which you can improve.

RESOURCES

Buchbinder, S. B., and J. M. Thompson. 2009. *Career Opportunities in Health Care Management: Perspectives from the Field.* Sudbury, MA: Jones & Bartlett.

Dye, C. F., and A. N. Garman. 2015. *Exceptional Leadership: 16 Critical Competencies for Healthcare Executives,* second edition. Chicago: Health Administration Press.

Goldsmith, M., with M. Reiter. 2007. *What Got You Here Won't Get You There: How Successful People Become Even More Successful.* New York: Hyperion.

Palmer, P. J. 2000. *Let Your Life Speak: Listening for the Voice of Vocation.* San Francisco: Jossey-Bass.

Tyler, J. L. 2011. *Tyler's Guide: The Healthcare Executive's Job Search,* fourth edition. Chicago: Health Administration Press.

Master the Informational Interview

No matter where you are in your career—a seasoned veteran or someone who's just starting out—you can benefit from informational interviews. The practice has had a significant effect on my own professional life, enabling me to stretch my vision and understanding of the field and those who lead it in interesting and dynamic ways. Not only are informational interviews a great way to establish and expand one's network, they're a great way to meet mentors and future colleagues. Taking the time to understand others' perspectives has been a critical ingredient to my own professional success.

—*Bryan Arkwright,*
director, Center for Telehealth, Mission Health,
Asheville, North Carolina

WHETHER IT HAPPENS over coffee or across a conference table, whether striding side by side on a midmorning power walk or chatting between bites of a sandwich in a hospital cafeteria, the informational interview is an exceptional strategy for advancing your career. Such interviews offer a multitude of benefits because they allow you to meet new contacts, ask about job opportunities, attend industry events, and gather other perspectives about organizational problems and solutions. Such interviews also sharpen your understanding of who the key players are in your professional circle and broaden your appreciation of the ways healthcare organizations operate. Whether you're fresh out of graduate school and angling for a job or you hope to glean best practices by understanding other organizations' methodologies, informational interviews are a boon at any point in your career.

Although informational interviews may lack the pitch of a full-fledged job interview, they ought to be taken just as seriously even if the meeting feels casual. Informational interviews are a chance not only to be inquisitive but to show your very best self. Make sure that you seize the opportunity.

At the outset of your career, such interviews will happen naturally. When you're professionally more established, you'll need to be more active in arranging these types of meetings. Here are a few guiding concepts:

- **Take every informational interview seriously.** Prepare in advance, and be sure to review background information about the person you're meeting, the company where he or she works, and any new initiatives or strategies it has recently employed. Has the company been in the news? Has it recently released an earnings report or had difficulties with patient outcomes or profits? Know this information. It's part of being a good guest—and a well-prepared one.

- **Be determined but polite.** Make a list of ten people you'd like to meet who have positions in companies you find interesting. One by one, try to connect with them, remembering to be unfailingly polite as you establish contact. The goal is to engage a steady stream of meetings throughout your career.

- **Leverage your references.** When you share a mutual acquaintance with the person you're interested in meeting, they often feel a sense of obligation. "My uncle (professor, cousin, teammate) thought we should meet, and I'm interested in knowing more about you, your professional trajectory, and your company. Do you have an hour to meet?"

- **Be prepared to ask for what you want.** If someone asks, "How can I help you?" be prepared to give a well-thought-out answer. Expressing what you want in a couple of sentences may require preparation and take some practice, but you'll be glad you have this "elevator speech" in your back pocket.

- **Ask good questions.** Understand generally the job description of the person with whom you're meeting so that you can ask engaging, relevant questions. Know what the company does and whom it serves as well as some basic statistics about it (number of beds, number of patients, annual revenue, and the like). If you pose off-target questions, you'll be remembered as ill prepared and amateurish.

- **Be interested.** People love to speak about their own career trajectories—the paths they followed, the opportunities they had, and the challenges they faced—and if you appear bored or disengaged, you're not only being rude, you're also leaving a bad impression. Ask good questions, make eye contact, nod while they're talking, and be a good, engaged listener.

- **Be thoughtful.** Meet with people at all levels and in all areas, not just in the C-suite. You can learn from successful people everywhere.

- **Remember the time.** Limit your meeting and questions to the amount of time allotted for the interview. Keep track of the time, and when you're getting close to the end of the hour, tell your interviewee that you wish to be respectful of his time, thereby acknowledging that it is precious.

- **Be grateful.** Be sure to write a handwritten thank-you note promptly after the meeting, and thank any assistants who helped you set it up. Within 24 hours of your interview, send a LinkedIn invitation to your interviewee to keep connected.
- **Keep it going**. As you meet with people, keep refreshing your list of ten by adding someone new. Continue this activity throughout your career.

So how do you get the conversation going? Ask open-ended questions that aren't too bland or general, such as the following:

- When you were first beginning your career, what did you see as your ultimate job?
- What things did you do early on in your career that influenced the way you think and do your job today?
- What do you like best about the company where you work?
- What's most difficult about your job there?
- What's your advice to someone like me? What should I be reading, thinking about, or doing to get perspective on the field?
- Are there other people whom you think I should meet with?

Though your approach will be informed by where you are in your career, don't be afraid to ask pointed (but polite) questions about practices at your interviewee's company. Be prepared to offer helpful suggestions to show you've been paying attention. "I noticed that you are promoting diabetes awareness in your advertising," you might say to the hospital's vice president of marketing. "We recently had a health awareness project in graduate school that has given me some ideas on the subject." Be succinct and positive. Your ideas might capture their attention—along with your motivation and poise.

While it's best not to convey your perspective with swagger, even fresh out of graduate school and early in your career you may have more ideas to offer than you think. Smart executives are interested in hearing new ideas from all sources and will value the opportunity to talk to someone who's smart, conveys information readily, and has plenty of innovative solutions.

If feasible, stay engaged with the person you're interviewing even after the interview. For example, if you mention a reference you found compelling, the interviewee might say, "Could you please send me that article?" If this type of interaction takes place, be sure to follow up immediately.

EXERCISE 1

Make a list of people who have jobs you find interesting and about whom you want to learn more. Develop a plan to request informational interviews. The best advice about advancing your career may come from someone who has a job you think you would like.

EXERCISE 2

Develop a one-page document after the interview that records what advice and perspective you were given. Include as much contact information as possible, including the correct spelling of the interviewee's name, his or her title, e-mail addresses, assistant's name, and so on. Use this information to stay in contact with this new person in your network.

If you especially liked the interviewee's job, field, position, or organization, note this information in your professional development plan (see Lesson 41). It will be useful in identifying the people or organizations you want to target when the time comes to apply for a new job or establish a new initiative.

RESOURCES

Alboher, M. 2008. "Mastering the Informational Interview." *The New York Times.* Published January 29. http://shiftingcareers .blogs.nytimes.com/2008/01/29/mastering-the-informational -interview/?_php=true&_type=blogs&_r=0.

Neil, J. 2014. *Informational Interview Handbook: Essential Strategies to Find the Right Career and a Great New Job.* New York: New Career Breakthrough.

Know and Use Your Strengths

Knowing your strengths doesn't always mean being strong. As you work with peers, colleagues, and subordinates, you will be called upon to be empathetic and human in the midst of making strategic decisions. The human side of leadership, which is a valuable asset, requires development and practice. This skill is portable and can be taken with you as you pursue new and different opportunities.

—*Ginger Cohen, MS, RN, FACHE,*
oncology program director,
Plaza Medical Center of Fort Worth, Texas

WHAT *REALLY* GETS you out of bed and amped up to work in the morning? What parts of your job do you sing (rather than slog) your way through? What professional domains *really* catch your interest?

Learning your strengths and using them effectively is key to success in any field, healthcare included. Strengths might be things that you're good at or that you enjoy—but ideally they're both. They can be overarching qualities ("I like assuming the helm of a project") or smaller and more task oriented ("I like creating spreadsheets"), but they should be *yours*. Identifying what you're good at and how you like to spend your time comes first.

There was a time when people thought that working on weaknesses was the best way to become a well-rounded professional.

But it's the reverse that's really true. Knowing your strengths will be an advantage throughout your career.

Once you identify what you're good at, do those things as often as you can. Surround yourself with people whose own strengths complement yours, not people who are carbon copies of you and your assets. If you're a great leader but are weak in finance, for example, aim for a leadership position and learn to recruit talented professionals who can support and oversee the organization's finances. If you're better at behind-the-scenes activities and prefer to keep your nose to the grindstone working on tasks rather than on big, messy, visionary projects with few parameters, acknowledge this about yourself. There is no shame in or advantage to either. So own the skin you're in—you'll be happier in the long run being yourself.

That said, don't expect your job to relentlessly please you once you've identified your favorite tasks—no job offers constant fun. Just know how to relish the time you do spend doing things you love.

So how do you know what you're good at? Here are a few questions to get you started:

- What do you get excited about doing?
- When you've been successful, what specific strengths did you tap?
- What do others say you're good at?
- What's been revealed to you in your performance reviews?
- How do your customers, patients, or clients view you?
- Do you see a difference between what you like doing and what you're good at? Or are they the same?

Some professionals keep a journal, listing projects they've worked on and what enabled their success. If you rate each project on a ten-point scale, you'll likely reveal what personal gifts you used en route. Others undergo formal analyses (e.g., the Myers-Briggs assessment, the VIA Survey) to identify their tendencies and assets. Still others tap professional coaches, who can help identify strengths and address weaknesses.

A few remarks:

- **Beware of thinking you will be perpetually weak in an area given early negative experiences.** People change and grow, honing and developing skills over the course of their lives. Just because you were a rotten math student, as so many people profess, doesn't mean you will always be bad at finance. Some deficits can be addressed with education and practice, and as a result, some things you consider weaknesses may actually become strengths. Don't simply assume that your weaknesses are cast in cement because of your past.

- **Don't get lazy with your strengths.** Just like regular exercise, your strengths need to be used regularly to ensure their fitness. Don't simply assume you'll always be good at something if you never practice it or don't seek out tasks to stretch and further cultivate what you're good at. Keep those asset muscles toned.

- **Develop an elevator speech.** Learn to describe your greatest strengths in two to three sentences so that you'll be prepared to introduce yourself and convey your skills to influential people quickly and competently without braggadocio. Assert your assets, and own them comfortably and well. If the CEO of your company got on the elevator with you, and you had two floors to tell her about yourself, what would you say? *Know this in advance.*

You can follow these tips merely by taking the time to know yourself. Once you've done that, you'll use your strengths to your advantage—just by knowing what they are.

EXERCISE 1

Keep a journal, listing projects you've worked on. List the strengths you used and the outcome of each project. As you review your journal, look for patterns. What role did you play in your most successful projects? Were you the leader, or did you serve in another capacity? Studying your own track record will give you a good indication of where your true strengths lie.

EXERCISE 2

Prepare an elevator speech describing your greatest strengths in two to three sentences. Then practice your elevator speech with your mentor or friends. Practice makes perfect!

RESOURCES

Buckingham, M., and D. O. Clifton. 2001. *Now, Discover Your Strengths.* New York: The Free Press.

Rath, T. 2007. *StrengthsFinder 2.0.* New York: Gallup Press.

Choose Your Mentor

Regardless of the stage of our career, we have mentors all around us. They're the people in the positions we aspire to achieve, the peers at our side, and those we lead. And each of us, regardless of the stage of our career, is an example for others around us. In a formal mentor relationship, I look for the protégé to be willing to listen, ask good questions, describe stumbles or tough spots, spend quality time thinking about the feedback received, and not expect the mentor to be the source of a future job. Ultimately, the key contribution of the protégé is to take ownership of the relationship.

—*Major General David A. Rubenstein, FACHE,*
US Army, retired

EACH OF US is the product of a variety of influences. Consider the people you've crossed paths with during your life who have exerted an influence on you: Your family, teachers, coworkers, and friends have all made their mark on your personality, perspective, aspirations, and work ethic. What lessons you take away from others and the way you synthesize and internalize what others say and do by mimicking it (or moving far away from it) shape who you ultimately become, how effectively you work, and, in many ways, how successful your career is.

But unlike your family, friends, and teachers—who were essentially assigned to you—you might *actively* choose professional mentors for a number of reasons, especially early on in your career.

Professional mentors are those whom *you* choose in the business world to impart advice, share knowledge, and serve as sounding boards. They can help you widen your network, review your résumé, and coach you as you prepare for an interview. The best mentors always take your calls and give you an honest opinion. Your mentor does not have to be in exactly the same field as you or even in a job that you consider to be your dream gig. Most important is to find someone who has traits you admire and seek to have—and someone with whom you feel comfortable.

In the mentor–mentee relationship, the formality of the arrangement is up to you. You do not need to declare someone your mentor so much as to connect with him or her on a regular basis, communicating about issues that concern you, deficits you perceive in yourself, and problems you're having at work. They will likely be flattered that you consider them a guide, however casual the arrangement is.

Others may feel more comfortable establishing a regular meeting schedule with their mentors, defining expectations, and charting a path of focus. Some mentors and mentees even work out the terms of their relationship on paper to keep themselves organized and honest. The parameters of schedule and relationship are entirely up to you and your mentor.

The key is to snag the opportunity when it presents itself. And sometimes that happens unexpectedly. If you meet someone you like who shows an interest in your career, you might ask, "Would you be willing to mentor me for the next few months while I try to improve my leadership skills?" or "Will you help me with my job search? I seem to be having problems during interviews." Most mentors are glad to pay it forward for help they received over the course of their own careers, and they feel organically happy to help an ambitious young professional eager to learn. Being a good student is the best way to show gratitude to your mentor. So is determining to be a mentor yourself when the opportunity presents itself down the line.

So whom do you tap, and how?

- You might retain a long-term relationship with a former professor or boss.
- Peers often make excellent mentors, especially if they have facility in a certain domain that you lack.
- People whose professional fields touch yours tangentially can offer a valuable perspective or a way of thinking that you otherwise might not have considered.
- Senior executives who have just retired make great mentors because they often have a lot of experience as well as the time and inclination to help.
- Colleagues who have three to five years' more experience than you are ideal because they have just traveled the path that you hope to take.

Occasionally, more formal routes to choosing a mentor are available. Some universities, trade associations, and companies have mentoring programs that pair seasoned executives with new ones. But not everyone has a pool of appropriate mentors from which to choose, and if you've determined that you need a mentor, it may be up to you to find one.

If you sense a scarcity of qualified casual mentors around you, you might consider investing money in hiring a career coach. Coaches—paid professionals, often certified—are another route to developing your best self and making good decisions. A "mentor for pay" can be useful in all the ways more casual mentors can be, but they often have the benefit of a particular perspective on a certain field, such as healthcare, and may prove to be an excellent investment during a difficult job search or transition. You also have the benefit of reliable accessibility, given that it's a service you're paying for.

Whatever the arrangement, understand that *you* are responsible for the bulk of the work. You're tapping a source, whether you're paying for it or not and whether it's formally agreed upon or casual, so be ready to take on the more active role. Arrange regular meetings with your mentor, and stay in touch by phone and e-mail. When you need help, ask for it—but always be respectful of your mentor's time.

You will need mentors throughout your career, so be sure to nurture and maintain these relationships even after the bulk of the mentoring has transpired. Don't dump people after they've helped you; remember them, respect them, and recall the messages they gave you. Send them periodic notes long after regular contact has subsided. Remind them that they served a critical function in your career and that you owe them your gratitude—and much else besides. Your thoughtfulness will, most likely, be more than enough thanks for them.

EXERCISE 1

Make a list of people who have mentored you during your personal and professional life, and list the issues they've helped you deal with. If you can't think of anyone, consider the work colleagues who might have provided you with advice and perspective about a specific issue.

EXERCISE 2

Draft a written statement about what you hope to gain from your mentor. Make a formal agreement, and use it with your mentor.

RESOURCES

Dye, C. F., and A. N. Garman. 2006. "Mentors: How to Identify, Approach, and Use Them for Maximum Input." Appendix C in *Exceptional Leadership: 16 Critical Competencies for Healthcare Executives.* Chicago: Health Administration Press.

International Coach Federation. 2014. "Coaching with Distinction." http://coachfederation.org.

Jenkins, C. Y., J. S. Lindsey, and J. Andrews. 2014. "Mentoring: A Tool for Building Your Career." www.box.net/shared /e4bxa219ad.

Develop a Professional Development Plan

It's easy to get caught up in the day-to-day hustle and bustle of a job, as you strive to achieve the objectives in your current position, but taking the time to develop a PDP is a priceless investment in your career. Begin by thinking about your passions, what constitutes your dream job, and the road map it takes to get there. Once you have developed your PDP, make a habit of reviewing it a few times a year, ideally with a trusted mentor. This is a great opportunity to be certain you're following your road map. And while it may need to be tweaked over time, a focused approach will ensure you stay on track to achieve your short- and long-term goals.

— *Leigh T. Sewell,*
chief of staff and vice president, children's services,
Bon Secours Virginia Health System, Richmond

IT'S EASY, ESPECIALLY early in your career, to cast about aimlessly and let the world happen *to* you. Many young careerists, unsure of their direction, end up wasting valuable time and effort in this manner. But absence of a decision is still a decision. With a bit of focus and planning at the outset of your professional life, you can reap the rewards down the line. And the best place to begin that focus is with a professional development plan (PDP).

Developing a PDP or career plan—essentially a map of your desired professional trajectory—is one of the most important ways you can harness direction. The plan itself doesn't have to be long, fancy, or formally written or contain more than a few pages of notes that mean something to you. The important thing is to take the time to consider your strengths and hopes, jot them down, and then regularly revisit them every year or so as you move into your chosen profession, pivot between jobs, undertake key assignments, or determine a new interest or direction. You might be surprised how dramatically your situation can change in just a few short years.

Steve recalls conducting a mock interview for a very green, very fumbling first-year master's of health administration student who repeatedly twirled and dropped his pencil. The student's PDP asserted that he wanted to be a hospital CEO within a decade—a plan that, at the time, seemed hard to imagine. Today, however, seven years after graduate school, he's not only a successful hospital CEO, but he also says he owes his success to having a plan he stuck to.

A PDP will help you identify the skills and passions you have. Knowing these will, in turn, enable you to decide what sort of job is a strong match for your skills. And although no absolutely perfect job exists, having a plan helps you step toward the best possible opportunities for you. The earlier in your career you can identify what you want out of your professional life, the better.

PDPs aren't only useful on paper. If you're able to verbalize the things that really excite you, your mentor, friends, or colleagues might be able to offer perspective about what they see in you and suggest ideas, job prospects, and companies that are a prudent match for you. Hearing what others say and perceive about you can be just as valuable as knowing what enlivens your mind and sustains your interest. So take the time to talk about your professional goals with others, and then listen to what they say. The best mentors will hear you, process the information, and offer you perspective about your best trajectory—and possible next steps.

Begin crafting your PDP by jotting down the answers to these questions:

- **What gifts and skills do you possess?** These gifts and skills can be difficult to ferret out on your own, so ask your parents, mentors, friends, supervisors, and colleagues to help you identify them. Early careerists might take personality tests, such as the Myers-Briggs assessment, to reveal their strengths, traits, and predilections. Some executives find it helpful to keep a personal project journal that details work successes to identify what issues they've tackled with poise and precision. If you've got a job or two under your belt, consider jotting down some notes about a few projects that have meant something to you, what you liked about them, and why they succeeded. A task that offered you a taste of a certain area of work that you ended up enjoying is sometimes enough to reroute an entire career path. Pay attention to what you've particularly enjoyed tackling in your job.
- **Where are your deficits?** Are you too fussy, or are you not detail oriented enough? Are you disorganized? Are you overly sensitive? What skills do you need to hone? Create a personal to-do list.
- **What are you passionate about?** Just knowing what you *can* do or are good at isn't enough; determine what really excites and engages you. Are there volunteer positions that have captured your imagination? People with whom you'd be thrilled to work? Certain types of initiatives that deeply interest you? In your ideal world, are you a teacher, an explorer, a researcher, a storyteller—or all of the above?
- **How did you get where you are?** Review your work history, the timeline of what you've done over your career. What were your significant turning points? Who played significant roles?
- **What's your ideal job?** Make a list of positions you'd want to pursue. Do these jobs require additional training

and education? More years of experience? Is any particular job feasible at the moment or a long-term goal?

- **Where do you want to live?** Have you considered living abroad? Are there states or regions you love—or places you'd *never* want to live? Or are you determined to keep to a particular zip code, sticking close to family and friends? Understand your practical professional parameters, and remember that while limiting your geographic area is fine, you may also be limiting your opportunities.

- **What are your target companies?** If there are dream jobs, there are dream companies too. As part of your PDP, list between a dozen and 20 organizations you admire in which you would want to work. Learn more about each prospective employer. Read up on the people who populate the organization as well as their backgrounds, experience, and education levels. Ask others what they've heard about the place. Get a sense of its flavor, its mission and vision, and its history. As you gather facts, the company may come off your list—or move up to the top.

Put as much effort as you can into your PDP, but remember that it's not a showpiece like a résumé or a curriculum vitae; it's a practical document that's as fluid, alive, and dynamic as you are. Let *it* focus *you*. Having a PDP road map will help you achieve a career at the intersection of your gifts and your passions.

EXERCISE 1

Create a PDP using the questions above.

EXERCISE 2

Ask a colleague to create a leadership practice inventory about you based on what he or she observes in you. At the same time, complete the instrument yourself. Did your perceived strengths and weaknesses mesh?

RESOURCES

Dye, C. F., and A. N. Garman. 2015. "Sample Self-Development Plan." Appendix B in *Exceptional Leadership: 16 Critical Competencies for Healthcare Executives,* second edition. Chicago: Health Administration Press.

Scivicque, C. 2011. "Creating Your Professional Development Plan: 3 Surprising Truths." *Forbes.* Posted June 21. www .forbes.com/sites/work-in-progress/2011/06/21/creating-your -professional-development-plan-3-surprising-truths/.

Build Your Résumé

Résumés are merely facilitation tools to get you to the interview, so be careful about spending a great deal of time preparing a perfect document. Your real emphasis should be on networking. If you can get your résumé grade up to a C, you have done what you need to do—at that point you need to move on to and focus on networking. Remember: "Network, or not work!"

—J. Larry Tyler, FACHE, FHFA, FAAHC, CMPE,
chairman and CEO, Tyler & Company,
Atlanta, Georgia

A RÉSUMÉ'S SOLE purpose—it's *only* reason for existing—is to get you an interview with a prospective employer. And given the weight of its single, critical role, you'd be wise to put some degree of thought, effort, and creativity into it. Your résumé should succinctly tell your story *and* clearly demonstrate how you can help employers solve the problems they're experiencing. Both of those components are equally important.

But before all that, consider what you need to do to get the kind of job you want. As you accomplish the tasks needed to achieve your professional goals, be sure to include those skills on your résumé as experience, education, and accomplishments. As you map out that plan on paper, in your mind, and verbally with others, you should find that you've got a lot of bragging points.

Here are a few tips as you create or revisit your résumé:

- **Consider its style.** As with dress, writing, and oral presentation, style matters. The historical résumé—a format that offers a timeline tally of your education, professional experience, accomplishments, skills, and awards in chronological order (most recent first)—is the résumé style most commonly used in healthcare. This kind of résumé is what most employers are looking for. If you've got a curriculum vitae–style résumé, as most academics and physicians do, consider reformatting it if you're interviewing for an executive or management position. Even if you're a physician executive, use the historical style. Anything else will feel dissonant and possibly opaque to your interviewers. It also may mean that the interview door remains tightly shut. Keep it accessible.

- **Quantify your work and results.** Populate your résumé with work that achieved measurable results. If you're not currently doing work that's quantifiable in some way, volunteer for such projects. Doing so will reap dividends when it's time to update your résumé. Have you helped reduce a hospital's infection rate? Led initiatives in diabetes education and nutrition counseling in the community? Improved customer service? Supervised a large staff, engaged in populating certain staffing areas, or overseen national research grants as part of your job? If so, quantify what you've done. Consider the power of saying, for example, that you've "led a project that reduced hospital infection rates by 5 percent over two years." Figure out how to capture your work in this way—and capitalize on it.

- **Use action words.** You didn't just have a staff of 30; you *led* a staff of 30 direct reports. You weren't just responsible for sales, nurse hires, or imaging; you "increased sales by 15 percent over the previous year," "spurred an 8 percent growth in imaging volume between 2013 and 2014," and "recruited two dozen nurses to populate eight units, bringing each unit up by 25 percent and to proper staffing levels."

Consider these points, too:

- You need only one résumé, so don't spend a huge amount of time crafting different résumés for different positions that highlight and showcase different talents. The majority of your time is best spent networking.

- You don't need to state a career objective in your résumé—you can do so in a cover letter or during an interview. Remember that the purpose of the résumé is to provide a profile snapshot. More critical is how you leverage your network so that your résumé gets funneled to the right person and lands you that interview.

- Always keep your résumé to a single page, adding a second page only after you gain considerable experience. More important than its length is covering the most important points concisely.

- Include all of your jobs in chronological order, starting with the most recent. Jobs you held more than ten years ago and temporary work may be listed without detail. If you worked several jobs during college, you can group them together.

- List the dates (month and year) of your education and graduation, your major and minor, and any honors. Your degree should be listed *exactly* as it is on your diploma. For example, if you earned a master of science degree in health administration but your diploma says only "master of science," that is what you put on your résumé—not "MSHA," a term that can be tricky or confusing.

- Don't forget to list internships, fellowships, and research you've assisted with, especially if you're an early careerist.
- Provide three to five bullet points for each work entry. Emphasize your most recent experience by including more detail. Your prospective employer will look most closely at and be most interested in what's happened lately. For each entry, balance responsibilities with accomplishments that can be quantified. Ask yourself the questions "How did I add value?" and "What will I be remembered for?" Your work entries should not read like a job description!
- *Never* attach a picture to your résumé.
- *Never* overstate your role or accomplishments. If you were a summer intern and helped design an orientation program for new physicians, do not say that you were in charge of new-physician orientation.
- Make sure your résumé has absolutely perfect spelling and grammar. Even if it makes you feel awkward, have someone whom you trust proofread your résumé for errors. Errors = no interview. Don't embarrass yourself—be sure it's right.

Everyone has a unique opinion about résumés, interviews, and cover letters—but know that no matter what, the classic approach is best. Beware of asking too many people for advice or heeding oddball recommendations to get noticed in an ocean of applicants. In the end, who and what you are—and where you come from—will be your best selling points. Your résumé gets the door open a crack; the rest is all you.

EXERCISE 1

Pull out the résumé that you completed in college or for your last job interview, and update it.

EXERCISE 2

Ask someone to critique your résumé and to give you feedback on ways to improve it.

RESOURCE

Tyler, J. L. 2011. *Tyler's Guide: The Healthcare Executive's Job Search,* fourth edition. Chicago: Health Administration Press.

Network Like You Mean It

It's not what you know, whom you know, or how popular you are; it's about building relationships with professionals who can speak to your abilities, performance, and skills as an emerging leader. Relationship building and networking, both inside and outside your organization, are crucial during your career. Identify mentors who are trustworthy, transparent, and authentic with you as well as those who will challenge your critical thinking and business acumen. Join professional organizations, such as the American College of Health Executives (ACHE) and the National Association of Health Services Executives, to learn more about the industry's best practices through your colleagues and mentors. And above all, take risks, differentiate yourself, and never subscribe to the absolute norm. Be memorable and always be yourself.

—Quinnetta Claytor,
performance improvement manager,
HCA Corporate Group,
Nashville, Tennessee

THE TERM *NETWORKING* is commonly used in business for good reason: Everyone grasps its importance. What's less clear is exactly *how* to build a network, *how* to expand it, and *how* to maintain it. Many mistakenly assume that those with strong networks are simply lucky, unfailingly popular, and easygoing; that socializing is a breeze for them; and that they can work a room with poise and ease.

For most of us, networking is indeed hard work. But as a tool to find your next job, advance your career, and meet other like-minded people, nothing is more important—and often, nothing is more satisfying.

And it's impossible to underestimate the criticality of networking. Roughly eight in ten people land healthcare executive jobs through effective networking. And as you progress up the career ladder, you'll have (and require) a larger network of professional relationships on which to rely.

So what is networking? It's simply establishing mutually beneficial professional relationships. And often, the most effective way to begin a networking relationship is to offer yourself in service to others. Can you tell someone about a job opening? Can you provide a reference? Do you have a particular perspective or experience with a company or client? Can you link two people together who have similar career trajectories? If you're helpful to others first, you'll likely be remembered for your kindness and connectivity—and your relationships will have a high chance of success and longevity. People remember those who have helped them professionally. And perhaps, down the line, you can be on the receiving end of the relationship—getting important job advice, obtaining a reference, hearing about an open position, or being able to initiate a meeting with a mutual colleague.

Networking has four basic components: building, organizing, growing, and maintaining the network.

- **Build it.** Each of us already has some kind of a network, even if many of us don't recognize it—so no one will be starting completely from scratch. Consider your family, friends, neighbors, classmates, teachers, clergy, and business associates. Consider fellow members of clubs, alumni groups, trade associations, and church congregations. Recall former coworkers and employees, or those of your spouse or partner. Tap your children's friends' parents or those you know through the local schools.

Then consider people outside your existing circles. Do you know anyone who might know successful people you would like to meet in your target field? Might casual links through friends, family, and coworkers enable you to set up a meeting or informational interview with someone at a company you admire? You might tell your neighbor you're hoping to launch a career in healthcare administration. "Do you know anyone," you could ask, "who could help me learn about the field?" Let that be your refrain.

- **Organize it.** Use LinkedIn and other social media sites as a way to follow connections with those you know, those you'd like to know, companies that interest you, and those in your field. Read trade publications to learn about job transitions and promotions. Keep your contact list and network database clean and up to date; when you hear of a change, record it immediately. Keeping this information updated and accurate is critical.

- **Grow it.** People often focus on expanding their networks when they're hunting for a job but then stop reaching out once they've landed one. That's a mistake. Think of networking like regular exercise—and always pay attention to it throughout your career. Connect online with those you've just met, and then stay connected via e-mail (sending interesting articles or congratulations on job anniversaries or new consulting gigs) and occasionally in person. Routinely tap people in your network with the question, "Who else should I be meeting?"

And remember the value of volunteering. Participation in trade organizations is a great way to fortify your network and meet like-minded individuals. Offer to speak at an upcoming meeting, or write articles for a trade-group newsletter. As you grow your network, however, remember to be both discreet and sensitive to your current employer. Do not meet with competitors in your market. So whereas talking to a former classmate at a local ACHE reception is acceptable, meeting with the CEO of a competitor organization in a networking capacity is not appropriate.

- **Maintain it.** You can maintain your network by sending pertinent and interesting articles by e-mail and LinkedIn postings (but do this judiciously, taking care not to become one of those who constantly forward e-mails), writing quick but thoughtful notes, making phone calls, and occasionally meeting in person. Remember which topics those in your network find meaningful: "Mr. Jones," you might write, "I am sending you this article because I remember that you said you were interested in developing a diabetes program at your hospital. I hope that you will find it useful. Do let me know if I can ever be of assistance."

Connecting with those in your network doesn't have to be a weighty, lengthy process. Suggest meeting your contacts for morning coffee before work, a quick lunch, or a connection at a local industry event. Set a goal of meeting someone in your network and outside your workplace at least once a month using the informational interview tactic described in Lesson 38. Be sure to include contacts from companies outside your current employer. Talk shop, and ask questions. Discuss problems you're facing, and ask for opinions.

EXERCISE 1

The next time you attend a reception or function, look at the list of attendees and identify people you'd like to meet. Learn as much as you can about the organizations represented by attendees and the reasons people are attending the event. Arrive early, and do your best to meet the people who you think can help you. As you meet people, ask for their contact information, give them yours, and contact them soon after the reception with a quick note.

EXERCISE 2

Update the contact information of people in your network. Make a list of people that you would like to add to your network.

RESOURCE

LinkedIn. 2014. "HealthCare C-Suite" (group). www.linkedin .com/groups/HealthCare-CSuite-3881687.

Interview Well (Part I)

Research, research, research! Learn everything you can about the organization, the industry, and the individuals with whom you'll be interviewing. There's absolutely no replacement for it.

—*James C. Godwin Jr., SPHR,*
vice president of human resources,
Bon Secours Virginia Health System, Richmond

LIKE MANY THINGS in life, a successful job interview begins with good preparation. You should prepare for an interview as you would prepare for a big game or an important test: with focus, organization, and precision. Consider your personal stories, what motivates you, and what makes you a strong candidate. Imagine several lines of questioning and the answers you'd provide. Try to figure out why and how you're a solid match for the company you may be working for.

Here are some helpful tips:

- **Know what you're getting into.** Be sure you know what format the interview will take: Is it with a group or a single person? Will you be having several brief meetings or one long one? Ask how long a meeting you should plan for—not by blurting "How long will this take?" but by inquiring discreetly and politely—and put aside at least twice that much time by clearing your calendar well before and after what's expected. If you can, get a sense of how formal the interview will be.

- **Do your homework.** Before the interview, research the company and its people. Has the company been in the news? Has it recently reported earnings or experienced a public snafu? Has it struggled with any high-profile safety or quality issues, and has it hired anyone important you should have on your radar? Has it expanded—or contracted—in recent years? Don't walk in knowing next to nothing about the place. Invest time in learning about the place and the people.

- **Get ready to ask smart questions.** Write down what you want to know about the position, the company's culture, the people you'd be working for, the people you'd be working with, and so on. Beware of asking questions that are vague or presumptuous—for example, "What's the culture like here?" or "How many vacation days will I get?"—because such questions can come across as rude or completely canned. Make your questions smart. For example, "Why do you think this problem happened after the merger took place?" or "I read about how that program thrived. How did your team make it such a success?"

- **Be ready for the old standby questions "Tell me about yourself" and "What is your greatest weakness?"** In response to the first question, give a full picture but limit it to three minutes or less. Share some facts—education, family, geography, and the like—but also explain what your plan is, what your general professional hopes are, and why you're interviewing there in particular (use your professional development plan as a rough guide). In response to the second question, be sure to explain how you're compensating for said weakness. If you say that you work too hard or that you're disorganized (two of the most clichéd answers, by the way, that you should avoid if you're able), talk about how you've learned a new software system that enables better filing, how you've taken up intramural soccer, or how you coach your kid's basketball team to achieve greater work–life balance. Good answers to these common questions show personal and professional awareness. Don't get tripped up by something so basic.

- **Know your stories.** Prepare eight to ten stories of two minutes or less that you can tap to answer behavioral questions, such as how you've used your leadership skills to solve problems at current or previous gigs. Use the S.O.A.R. method to frame your stories: a brief description of the *situation*, the *obstacles* you faced, the *action* you took, and the *results* you achieved. Be prepared to explain what you learned from problems you have faced in your career. For example, "I left my secure job at a large healthcare system to take a job at a startup company. Things did not work out there, but I learned the importance of innovation in healthcare."

- **Get perspective and clarity on salary.** Research what others in similar positions make, and be prepared to state your preferred salary (but only if asked) to show you've got a good idea of your worth. Don't hope for a pie-in-the-sky salary—stay within or close to the range of what people in similar positions make.

- **Maintain eye contact.** Don't stare, but gaze steadily. This usually gets easier a few minutes into the interview, once you're able to relax.

- **Bring extras.** Extra résumés, extra writing samples, extra materials from your portfolio, and extra paper and pencils to jot notes with—keep them neatly at the ready in case they're called for. If you're bringing a phone or computer with you, be sure it doesn't ring or chime at inopportune moments.

- **Be your best self.** Get a good night's sleep before the interview. Don't eat or drink excessively the evening before, and beware of foods that may have any lingering effects.

- **Know where you're going and how long it will take to get there.** There's nothing worse than getting lost or being late on interview day. Be sure you know where to report and what the parking situation is, and do a dry run by visiting the site beforehand. Observe how other employees dress, and take your cue from what you see.

- **Dress your best** (see Lesson 16). Conservative business dress is the order of the day. If you can afford it, purchase a new set of clothes to look and feel the part. Pay attention to the details—hair, shoes, fingernails, and accessories should all be neat and business appropriate. Look like you care—your effort will shine through.

Those who don't prepare don't win. Take it seriously—know what you're going to say and how you're going to say it well before you shake hands and introduce yourself.

EXERCISE 1

Write down eight to ten brief stories that illustrate how you have solved problems and handled difficult situations in the past. Keep them updated, and prepare new stories as you gain experience. Use the SOAR answer model to explain the situation, obstacles, action, and results.

EXERCISE 2

Conduct mock interviews with friends and counselors. Prepare a list of possible questions, and practice answering them. Don't try to memorize the answers—answer them naturally, based on your experience. Use the stories you prepared to answer some of the questions.

RESOURCES

Byham, W., with D. Pickett. 1999. *Landing the Job You Want: How to Have the Best Job Interview of Your Life*. New York: Three Rivers Press.

Job Interview Questions. 2014. "Ace Your Next Interview and Get the Job!" Accessed November 11. www.job interviewquestions.org/.

Powers, P. 2010. *Winning Job Interviews*. Franklin Lakes, NJ: Career Press.

Interview Well (Part II)

The importance of the interview cannot be overstated. It's game day or it's the big recital—time to be our best. And yet, I tell all of my candidates to remember to relax, be prepared, and stay focused on the process. Otherwise, the stress and pressure can derail you.

—*Carson F. Dye, FACHE,*
senior partner, Witt/Kieffer, Chicago

GOOD NEWS! YOU'VE taken time with your résumé, tapped your network contacts, done your research, and now you're in the enviable position of interviewing for a job you really want and believe you could flourish in. This is truly show time—and your chance to put your best foot forward.

Interview day is when all your preparation pays off, when you're able to energetically demonstrate your ability to add value to an organization and show how you'd lead, solve problems, and be a match, personality-wise, for the company. This is the next-to-last step before landing a job. *You're nearly there.*

But first, some basics to start you off right. The morning of the interview, be sure to do the following:

- **Arrive early.** Give yourself a chance to calm down on-site by waiting for a few minutes in the lobby or cafeteria. Go to the restroom, and check your appearance.

- **Be in the reception area at least five minutes early.** And don't be more than 20 minutes early. Don't plan so far ahead that you're sitting there for a half hour or longer. Early is good—*too* early is not.

- **Be on your best behavior.** Introduce yourself to everyone you meet, and do your level best to remember names. If you're not good at it, use some kind of mnemonic device to improve your recall. For example, if you meet someone named Mary who's wearing red, you can remember her name by telling yourself she's "maroon Mary."

Once you've entered the office or board room, remember the following:

- **Be flexible.** Interview styles vary from company to company. Be prepared for a casual encounter as well as a more formal one. Don't be thrown by a group interview or a schedule that seems to have you meeting everyone in the organization one-on-one—or, conversely, by one that is more anemic than you anticipated. Also, don't let anyone sense that you're rattled by a shift in format or an abrupt departure from what you were told to expect. You want to demonstrate that you're able to think on your feet.

- **Distribute eye contact.** If you're interviewing with a group, direct your gaze primarily at the person who asked the question, but sweep your eyes around the table so that everyone feels addressed. Note the body language of each interviewer and the dynamic in the room.

- **Be consistent—and consistently polite.** You may be asked to meet with multiple people over a short period of time. Be consistent in your answers to questions, because interviewers are likely to compare notes. Don't get flustered by having to answer the same question more than once or feel put out by having to repeat yourself.

As the interview gets under way, remember:

- **Begin with a nice, firm handshake.** No floppy, sweaty, or cold hands, if you can help it. Repeat the name of the person you've just met so it'll cement in your mind.
- **Let the interviewer show you where to sit.** Then wait to be seated until you're invited to do so.
- **Maintain good eye contact.** Use a friendly (but not staring) gaze, and let the interviewer know you're listening by occasionally nodding or murmuring *uh-huh* or *yes* as they speak.
- **Fight the urge to fidget.** Don't touch your face, fiddle with your hands, play with your hair, or jiggle your legs during an interview. You don't have to be as still as a corpse, but keep extraneous nervous movements under wraps.
- **Project energy and alertness throughout the interview.** *Never* yawn or look distracted or bored.
- **Don't accept a coffee or drink if offered one.** Accept only if you think it rude not to do so. You're not there to refresh yourself—and spills happen to the best of us.
- **Remember to pace your speech.** Avoid babbling, and pause thoughtfully prior to answering each question. *Never* interrupt an interviewer, and if you yourself are interrupted, take a moment to receive what is being said before replying.
- **Smile occasionally.** Doing so will project a sense of confidence and ease and will show that you're glad to be there under consideration.

What is the interviewer looking for?

- The meeting gives the interviewer a chance to evaluate you, to determine if you are the best candidate for the job, and to decide whether you'll be a productive, responsible, engaging, and motivated employee. Be prepared to explain why you want the job and why you're a good fit. Your answers should clearly demonstrate the skills you bring and how you'll add value.

- Chemistry matters. The feeling an interviewer gets while interacting with you can be more important than your answers to questions. Take cues by observing your interviewer's demeanor. Be an engaged, thoughtful listener and speaker. Be friendly, funny (if appropriate), and always interested. Ask good questions.

Give good answers to the questions asked:

- **Lob the pleasantries right back.** Interviewers often begin with small talk and may reference current events, sports, or the weather. They may ask where you grew up and went to school. Let the interviewer take the lead. Use this opportunity to find a connection with the interviewer to help you relax.

- **Get ready for the opening question.** Perhaps it'll be something like "Tell me about your background"—to which you should have a response that lasts less than two minutes. Be clear, and keep it short. Don't ramble or go off on tangents.

- **Listen to and understand the question that has been asked.** Then pause, consider the question, breathe, and relax as you begin to answer it.

- **Observe the interviewer's body language.** If she looks bored or distracted, wrap up what you're saying and wait for the next question.

- **If you don't understand a question, smile, breathe, and ask for clarification.** Don't get stuck. Answer everything to the best of your ability, and remember that interview questions usually have no right or wrong answers. The interviewer will be observing how you handle pressure.

- **Don't inquire about salary and benefits unless the interviewer broaches the topic.** Be prepared to state your preferred salary if asked, a number you've decided in advance to show you have a good idea of your worth. This is not the time to have unrealistic salary hopes—know what other people in similar positions make, and stay within or close to that range.
- **Use stories to demonstrate your competencies** (see Lesson 44). Be sure to have eight to ten such stories in your back pocket that you can tap.
- **Keep up your side of the back-and-forth.** An interview is like a seesaw. Be prepared to ask as many questions as you need to during the process to understand the nature of the position and the culture of the company. You don't have to save your questions until the end if relevant points during the interview provide opportunities to ask them.

And finish strong:

- Summarize, in a sentence or two, why you would be a good hire for the company. Remember to say that you're grateful for the chance to be considered and that you're excited about the opportunity. Let them know you're particularly interested in the job now that you've learned more about it and had a chance to meet the people you'll be working with. Add that you look forward to hearing about next steps.
- And before you leave, ask what those next steps will be. Do they hope to have someone in place within a few weeks? Within a few months? Can you take any additional steps to show your interest? Perhaps you'll feel comfortable saying, "May I phone or e-mail you next week?"

After the interview, remember to do the following:

- Give the interviewer a solid goodbye handshake.
- Thank the receptionist by name.
- Send handwritten thank-you notes to everyone you met, dropping them in the mail either the same day or the following morning—no later. Timing here counts, so do it promptly even if you have to stay up late to get the notes written.
- Jot down notes. With whom did you meet? Make sure you write down names and titles correctly. What recurring themes did you perceive? What do you think you did well, and what didn't go as smoothly as you'd have liked?

Interviewing shouldn't be terrifying, but being nervous shows that you care. Although practice and experience will mitigate such feelings to a certain extent, you should always feel some anxiety over an interview. If you don't feel a smidgen of nerves, consider why—perhaps it's not a job you're interested in, or perhaps you've become a bit overconfident—and then reconsider. Nervousness serves a purpose, and no one's beyond it.

EXERCISE 1

Research every organization where you will have an interview. Try to gain an understanding of its culture and interviewing approach.

EXERCISE 2

Practice interviewing with a friend or mentor. Your mentor should play the role of the hiring manager for the position you are pursuing.

RESOURCES

Cattelan, L. 2012. "The S.O.A.R. Answer Model." Human Resources.com posting. www.humanresources.com/491/the -soar-answer-model/.

Lehigh University. 2014. "S.T.A.R. Method for Behavioral Interviewing." Career Services website. Accessed November 11. http://careerservices.web.lehigh.edu/node/145.

Handle Failures and Disappointments

I'm in a perpetual state of self-reflection. At the end of the day on my commute home or as I'm getting ready for bed, I tend to cycle through what I might've done differently to be a better leader— how I could have addressed a tough question more effectively, interacted with a colleague differently, or engaged a constituent better. Even if these weren't marked failures to others, to me they're opportunities that, if acknowledged and reflected upon, might lead to greater success in the future. They're reminders that continuous improvement doesn't just apply to quality indicators, patient satisfaction scores, or the bottom line: Leaders at all levels of an organization must be thoughtful about their impact on it, too.

—*Carrie Owen Plietz, MHA, FACHE,*
CEO, Sutter Medical Center–Sutter Health,
Sacramento, California,
and 2010 recipient of the ACHE Robert S. Hudgens
Memorial Award for Young Administrator of the Year

IT GOES WITHOUT saying that you'll have failures and disappointments in your life—no human alive is untouched by adversity. You'll be at the helm of failed projects, miss opportunities, experience mishaps with colleagues and clients, lose jobs, and suffer a host of personal losses. It's just part of life.

Because problems in life are guaranteed, the bigger question is how you'll handle them. Will you blame others for issues beyond your control? Will difficulties scare you away from thinking creatively and from taking risks? Will they create undue fear and anxiety? Or will you learn and grow as a result of your failures? The most seasoned executives know that dealing with setbacks right away is one key to being a successful leader. When bad stuff happens, the most effective managers know how to handle difficulties in the moment and in the hours and days after, synthesizing what didn't work to strengthen their process of discovering what *does* work for tasks down the line.

The strongest people turn failures into opportunities, put the past behind them, and focus on their future direction. Some, like mindfulness guru Deepak Chopra, MD, distinguish between failure and setbacks: Setbacks are temporary and surmountable, whereas failure is a setback that leaves a scar and induces fear, anxiety, and—in the worst cases—inertia. Therefore, it's crucial not to let short-term setbacks manifest themselves as long-term failures. If you begin with that idea, you can overcome almost anything.

Often, the best salve is close at hand and involves keeping busy, moving, and engaged. In your healthcare role, you are part of a core group of individuals who help people in need—and that reminder alone is powerful motivation and inspiration when times get tough. If your professional life has become sodden with controversy or you're in the thick of a setback, you might turn to family or faith, but you could also work at a local free clinic or volunteer on a hospital unit that needs a hand. Bring yourself up by bringing yourself back to the core reason you do what you do—that alone can put you on a path to recovery.

Never believe you'll be stuck in a problem's chasm forever. Stay as positive as you can, focusing on today and what you can do to move forward. And don't forget to forgive yourself for making mistakes. Own your error, acknowledge it to others and out loud, and then forgive yourself. Remember to view yourself as worthy and successful no matter what is happening. Believe wholeheartedly that you'll find your route to recovery—and soon it will be true. No problems last forever.

Here are some ideas to temper failures and disappointments:

- **Keep expectations reasonable.** Not everything you do can or will be great. But if you're achieving all you set out to do, you've probably set the bar too low. Stretch to achieve more difficult goals, even if success isn't always in the bag. Difficult successes are much more satisfying than easy ones.

- **Get comfortable with risk** (see Lesson 2). Take on new tasks with the understanding that you may experience setbacks. If you're offered a job that is a stretch, don't count all the reasons you might get stuck—take it. You may do better than you expect and, despite mistakes, may learn a great deal. Most successful entrepreneurs assert that they derived their greatest success from what came *after* abject failure.

- **Analyze what happened.** Talk to your colleagues to get the whole picture, being sure to own your part in what went wrong. Is your skill set weak? Are your interpersonal skills lackluster? Are others not pulling their weight? Perhaps coaching, professional development, or education might improve your (or your colleagues') next try. If your deficits are offset by the talents of certain staffers, be sure to get their help on the next project. Great leaders surround themselves with people whose strengths complement their weaknesses.

- **Don't brood.** Take the "where to from here?" approach. Getting past failures can take time, but beware of spending weeks lamenting an outcome that's preventing you from moving on. At some point, it's imperative that you press on—changed, better informed, and ready for what's next.

- **Talk about it—but not endlessly.** You're not the first one to bomb a presentation before the board, to have a conflict with a boss, or to get fired. Discuss your disappointments with others. Plenty of colleagues and friends in your network have felt the same sorrows and frustrations—talk to them about it, but not forever. Know when you've talked it through—and move on.

- **Hire people who have tried hard and failed.** Smart managers examine applicants both on their own and in the context of their work. People who try and fail are braver and far better bets than those who have followed traditional paths, never taken risks, and earned easy successes as a result.

As you make your way out of the morass of a large problem, do your best not to repeat your mistakes. If you find yourself making the same errors repeatedly, you may need the help of a mentor or professional coach. But if you're thoughtful about your experiences and are able to tap your own reservoir of self-worth and value, you'll pull through a lifetime's worth of setbacks. There's not one of them that you won't be able to topple.

EXERCISE 1

Write down what you consider important in your life. Understanding who you are will help you deal with loss and failure.

EXERCISE 2

If something went wrong, whom would you turn to? Whom do you talk with about problems? Make a list of people in your support group.

RESOURCE

Chopra, D. 2013. "How to Protect Yourself from Failure." LinkedInarticle. Posted November 23. www.linkedin.com /today/post/article/20131123022336-75054000-how-to -protect-yourself-from-failure.

Balance Life and Work

I used to look at work–life balance as a seesaw that had to be—and could only be—balanced by including equal parts of work and personal activities. I soon realized that achieving true balance, yet maintaining a focus on career growth early on, lies in implementing a movable fulcrum.

—*Matthew D. Inama, MHA,*
pharmacy finance manager, Department of Pharmacy,
The Ohio State University Wexner Medical Center, Columbus

HEALTHCARE IS IMPORTANT work, and people's very lives are affected by the decisions we and our colleagues make. Given the profession's demands on our time and energy, it's important to think long and hard about your personal priorities and to strike a balance between life and work. Despite the rigors of the field, with a little effort you *can* achieve some degree of balance, if not equity.

Here are some questions to guide you as you consider a company or position:

- **Do you work to live or live to work?** Be honest with yourself: Are you looking for a professional challenge, or do you want stability and a paycheck?
- **What's most important to you?** Make an honest list tallying where work, family, and hobbies rank in your life. Is coaching your son's soccer team a top priority? What

about having solitary time with your dog in the park every afternoon? Do you need to continue competitive cycling or running to keep yourself sane? List it. Your career will likely require trade-offs, so knowing what ranks where is critical.

- **What's your family situation?** You won't have endless chances to attend your daughter's birthday celebrations, your kids' first recitals, or your son's kindergarten play—children grow up fast. And you'd be smart to have frank and open discussions about your career with your partner or spouse, especially if he or she has a good job or if the relationship would crumble if you're in the office too much. Your personal relationships should be far more important than your job—unless you want to look back on your career and see a string of losses.

- **What's the company culture?** If you're considering a job at a new organization, talk to people who work there to get an idea of whether it fits the work–life balance you seek. Is it a "get the job done and go home" kind of place? Or one that will require long hours because of staffing levels, innovations that have no charted path, and large projects and initiatives on the horizon? If you're willing to go for the latter, remember that the rewards may be large— but mainly professional. Consider what's best for you, especially if you have a family, partner, or lifestyle that requires dedicated time away from the office.

- **How much travel is involved?** Travel can have a real impact on your personal life and can cut into your ability to enjoy routine pastimes. Given that companies often underestimate the amount of time employees travel, it's up to you to get a full picture of what will be required. Remember to build in time to travel to and from airports and hotels and to change planes. Also consider that a one-hour meeting in another city just a quick plane ride away can turn into a three-day trip if inclement weather or a complication arises.

- **What about weekends and flexibility?** Companies that require significant travel or weekend work often allow some degree of reciprocal flex time, but as a manager, your presence in the office is likely needed. Some managers set the tone in their office by leaving consistently at 5 p.m., whereas others are the last to leave. Know that your patterns in the office will affect how others perceive your diligence and effort. Researchers have found that those who arrive and end their day early tend to be considered less hard-working than those who start later and stay late—even if the total number of hours worked is the same. If you consistently leave early to tend to children, a hobby, or a relationship, those who keep more traditional hours may look at you askance. The same goes for working from home. Early on in your career, expect to put in long days to gain experience, credibility, and the respect of your colleagues.

And consider these additional ideas to help you strike the right balance:

- **Learn to say no politely but firmly.** Many people commit to new tasks without really thinking about how it will affect their home life. Learn not to take on new obligations without talking it over with your family first. If you're already tapped out, shed or delegate another of your tasks before agreeing to take on a new one.
- **Trim your to-do list.** Review your commitments, and, if possible, eliminate activities that you do not enjoy or that someone else can tackle.
- **Dedicate time to unplug.** Disconnecting periodically will enable you to be present when you need to be (see Lesson

8 on mindfulness) so that you can truly engage with the task or people before you.

- **Work smarter.** Cut time wasters from your life (see Lesson 3). Don't flit from assignment to assignment in a disorganized, inefficient manner. Be organized, and keep an organized office (see Lesson 22). Make sure you understand assignments before you start them, and learn to batch errands so that you can cut down on the number of trips you take.
- **Be your own master.** Control your schedule to the extent you can.

You alone are responsible for finding the right work–life balance. And although companies and technology allow greater flexibility than ever before, nothing replaces true face time and long hours—especially when you're the manager, and especially early in your career. Working smartly and efficiently and dedicating time during your day when you can focus your full attention and efforts on nonwork activities are good places to begin. And if you set boundaries, your work colleagues will generally respect them. If not, it may be time for a change.

EXERCISE 1

Make a list of the activities that you least enjoy, and consider dropping them.

EXERCISE 2

Have regular meetings with your family. Discuss your work and what you value the most with your family on a routine basis.

RESOURCES

Groysberg, B., and R. Abrahams. 2014. "Manage Your Work, Manage Your Life." *Harvard Business Review* 92 (3): 58–66.

Mayo Clinic. 2012. "Work–Life Balance: Tips to Reclaim Control." Published July 12. www.mayoclinic.org/work -life-balance/art-20048134.

Sandberg, S. 2013. *Lean In: Women, Work, and the Will to Lead.* New York: Knopf.

Uscher, J. 2013. "5 Tips for Better Work-Life Balance." Web MD. Posted March 28. www.webmd.com/health-insurance /protect-health-13/balance-life.

Commit to Lifelong Learning

Learning is a lifelong journey—not a destination. I have been fortunate to know many great leaders and, without fail, the most effective are those who not only commit to their own development but invest in the development of others. In healthcare, no one can afford to stand still, and while a commitment to learning does not guarantee success, you certainly can't be successful without a passion to learn.

—Deborah J. Bowen, FACHE, CAE,
president and CEO,
American College of Healthcare Executives, Chicago

AT NO POINT in your career—or your life, frankly—should you feel that you've somehow learned it all. The best, most authentic leaders commit to a curriculum of lifelong learning throughout their careers to keep current and stay relevant. While your formal education provides you with a regimented knowledge base at the outset, the field of healthcare and medical management is in near-constant flux. That means many of your most critical lessons will happen naturally on the job as you contemplate and solve real-world problems.

But even the richest on-the-job experiences don't offer you everything you need to learn and grow. Seek help from mentors, coaches, and bosses to keep current and to turn any personal or educational deficits you have into strengths. And be dogged about consuming information wherever, whenever, and as regularly as you can. Only *you* can drive that.

Here are a few tips to guide ongoing learning:

- **Read avidly.** Keep reading material on your bedside table, in your briefcase, and in your bathroom. Invest in subscriptions to magazines and journals related to your field. Read at least two books and two professional journals every month. Discuss the books with those in your network who share your interests, being sure to get their book recommendations as well. The more you read, the richer your ideas will become.

- **Set goals for self-improvement.** Your focus on what to improve skills- and knowledge-wise will shift from time to time. You can always boost your competence in certain areas. An executive who is afraid to speak in public, for example, might improve her proficiency by joining a local Toastmasters club. She might then volunteer to speak at small events, churches, or social clubs. As she gains confidence, she might seek more challenging venues.

- **Keep going.** Once you have mastered a new skill, start anew. Have you conquered public speaking? Aim to become a better writer. Want to hone your business communication skills? Take a course in crucial conversations so that you've got strategies to tap when facing a difficult interaction with a colleague or direct report.

- **Keep abreast of current strategies.** Learn everything you can about quality improvement techniques, such as Lean and Six Sigma, and strategies used to reduce waste and solve problems. Attend training programs that can expand your skill set in identifying activities that aren't adding value to your organization.

- **Take others with you.** As you widen your knowledge and understanding of best healthcare business practices, include the right mix of colleagues and stakeholders who, together, can help you focus on a problem and solve it. If multiple colleagues might benefit from a course or retreat, invite them to attend such seminars together.

- **Aim to become an expert.** When a subject piques your interest, consume everything you can on the topic. Books, journal articles, websites, blogs—be a voracious consumer. Being intensely interested in a subject makes it easier to consume, digest, and share what you know.

- **Learn what others do.** Soak up what you can from those whose jobs are different from yours. For example, if a physician performs a new procedure, express curiosity and ask to observe. See what other companies are doing so that you can understand what their best practices are. You might be able to mimic their strategies back home.

- **Be professionally malleable.** Once upon a time, it was a straight shot from an administrative residency to hospital president by age 40, but today, because of growth and change, such a career trajectory is no longer the case. Consider different professional aspects of healthcare that might be outside your comfort zone. Having a breadth of knowledge is positive for career advancement. You might consider a lateral move or a position in a different organization or country to widen the scope of your understanding and experience. Stretch yourself, and take on assignments you might never have imagined for yourself. Take a job that you know very little about, and master it. You'll be the better for it.

- **Affiliate with a professional association.** Organizations like the American College of Healthcare Executives, the Medical Group Management Association, or the Healthcare Information and Management Systems Society have a mission to improve the knowledge of members and offer venues for continuing education. Attend conferences and webinars, and read blogs. Join these organizations' social media and LinkedIn groups.

The bottom line? Don't sit still. The best future healthcare leaders are those who bring a rich variety of skills and experiences to the table and whose appetites for knowledge and growth are never satiated. Executives who have worked in multiple settings and who are professionally malleable will always be in high demand because they're flexible and can adapt quickly to new challenges. They are the people companies want—and need.

So even if it's out of your comfort zone, go for that gig in acute care, ambulatory care, medical group management, managed care, quality improvement, or finance. You'll learn a great deal about large and complex healthcare systems, you'll tackle issues you might never have imagined—and you and your career will be the better for it.

EXERCISE 1

In your professional development plan, you indicated gaps in your competencies and areas that need strengthening. Find continuing education opportunities or other ways to turn your weaknesses into strengths.

EXERCISE 2

Attend the American College of Healthcare Executives' Congress on Healthcare Leadership. Attend the Career Management sessions, and complete the instruments there that will help you develop a plan for lifelong learning.

RESOURCES

American College of Healthcare Executives. 2014. www.ache.org.

Healthcare Performance Partners. 2014. "Lean Healthcare Training." Accessed November 11. www.hpp.bz/lean healthcare/trainingservices.php.

Discern When It's Time to Leave

Leaving a job is tough, but if you have lost your enthusiasm and feel on edge because you have also lost interest, it's definitely time to go. Try not to look back and reminisce about the good old days; just get out gracefully, and get out fast. Wasting time in a negative situation drains your energy and enthusiasm as nothing else can. Get on with your career, and make the world your oyster. Don't make it more complicated than it is, and remember, when you leave any organization, do it with a smile on your face. Your positivity will pay dividends in the future—and it's the right thing to do.

—Charles S. Lauer, HFACHE,
speaker, adviser, writer, and former publisher
of Modern Healthcare *magazine*

HEALTHCARE IS EXPERIENCING tumultuous times, but change and financial challenges are hardly limited to our profession. *Every* manager should be prepared to change jobs numerous times during his or her career. And even if you love the job you're in, you should always have your hoped-for career trajectory and professional development plan in mind (see Lesson 41) and be open to opportunities that arise.

When it's time to go, always leave on the best terms possible. The world is small, and the person you rudely cut off in traffic today or speak disparagingly about to a friend might be your connection to your next big job. Never burn bridges.

An old adage quips, "It's better to leave six months too early than six months too late." The difficulty, of course, is knowing whether you've overstayed a job. Although you don't have to keep one foot out the door at all times, remain flexible and be prepared to move if things deteriorate beyond repair. Before you leave a job, evaluate your career plans, talk to your mentors and family, and carefully consider all of the factors that will affect your decision, including emotional and financial ones. And always remember that it is much easier to find a job while you still have one.

So how do you know when it's time to go? Consider these questions:

- **Why do you want to leave your job?** The answer should take less than two minutes to express, be on the tip of your tongue, and not require deep contemplation. Are your reasons rational, or are they emotional? Are you getting signs that it is time to go? Have you stopped learning new skills? Do you dread going to work every day? Are you receiving fewer invitations to key meetings, or have you stopped receiving them altogether? Do the negatives about your job outweigh the positives?

- **Do you feel consistently unhappy at work?** Life changes—for example, a birth, a death, a divorce, or a move—can sometimes spur professional discontent. Are you truly unhappy, or are you just in a funk? Is your current job the source of your unhappiness, or is it a mere bystander to it? Does work make you unhappy because of its time demands and excessive travel and because it separates you from your family? And if so, is it worth scrapping the entire job, or should you attempt to shift the way you do it?

- **Consider the effect changing jobs will have on your career.** Think about how it will look on your résumé. You do not want to be perceived as a job hopper. If you want to leave because you're having trouble meeting expectations, try to work through these problems—by doing so, you will learn and grow.

- **What will you do next?** You should have a solid concept of what comes next that you can articulate in two minutes or less.

- **How would changing jobs affect your family?** This question is important. Think practically. How does your spouse feel about you making a change? Can you sell your house? Where will you live? Will your partner need to get a job or work more hours to cover costs? Where will your children go to school? How important is living close to your extended family? Will the new position you seek require more travel and time away from home?

- **Are there solid reasons to stay?** Your current position should be part of your career plan and among the career goals you set for yourself to accomplish. Are there other unfinished goals that you can still attain in your current role? Have you expressed interest in a promotion, or do you know or sense you're on the shortlist for one? Does your name come up when your company has an opening?

- **Are you sure the change will be an improvement?** Some young executives leave a good position early on for a tantalizing increase in pay or because they felt undervalued, then find that they are worse off in the new position. Such pathways can derail your career. If something is not right in your current position, make your feelings known before you decide to leave. Discuss your situation with your boss and with the right people in human resources. State your concerns clearly—don't expect people to guess the source of your unhappiness. Explain what you think you need to be successful in your current role—you might be surprised how positively senior management responds.

Whatever the situation, your departure should be positive and professional. Be gracious when you're leaving a position—even if you've been fired—and do your best to leave on friendly terms. Healthcare is a smaller field than you might imagine, and you will likely cross paths with former colleagues time and time again.

And once you decide to leave, own your decision—don't look back or second-guess yourself. Every decision has degrees of good and bad. Over the course of our careers, we all end up in bad situations, in jobs that are a poor professional match, or in positions where we make mistakes. We're only human. But when one door closes, another one opens. Will you be ready for what's next?

EXERCISE 1

Keep your professional development plan (see Lesson 41) and your résumé (see Lesson 42) current, and make sure your network (see Lesson 43) is robust and up to date. If you were fired tomorrow, what would you do?

EXERCISE 2

Create a personal financial plan, and have enough cash to pay your bills for at least six months if you are not working.

RESOURCE

Tyler, J. L. 2011. *Tyler's Guide: The Healthcare Executive's Job Search,* fourth edition. Chicago: Health Administration Press.

Find Your Next Job

We all initially joined the healthcare field because it attracts noble, caring, and compassionate individuals—and occupies such a critical role in our society. So when it's time to head to your next job, always keep at the top of your mind not only what you've done but also what you do really well, and why. Be able to express these ideas to prospective employers as well as how your values— personal and professional—complement those of the organization. Above all, keep your chin up and your nose to the ground so you don't miss opportunities to find meaningful work and contribute to society. Looking for work is difficult, and rejection can be hard, but there is a job for everyone and it's the determined who ultimately find the roles that are most significant to their objectives.

—*Bo Cofield, DrPH, FACHE,*
associate vice president, hospitals and clinic operations,
University of Virginia Medical Center, Charlottesville

AN IMPORTANT PART of *any* successful career is the ability to find and transition into a new job when the time comes. Many executives have made successful moves that ignited their careers. Others rely on a series of lateral moves before breaking into the upper echelons of their profession. If you've established a robust network and acquired the range of skills you need to take your work life to the next level, your chances for success will be much higher.

A successful job search has several key ingredients:

- Plan and focus.
- Project confidence, and keep a positive attitude.
- Define your brand, and know what sets you apart.
- Keep a daily activity level that is consistent with your situation. If you do not have a job, your full-time job is to find one.

In the event you are terminated, you may need time to emotionally process the experience before refocusing your efforts on searching for a new job. Most people need time to grieve after they are fired, particularly if they held a position for a long time, and won't be ready to move on until they've come to terms with the loss. If your every thought begins with how you were professionally mistreated, you likely haven't gotten over it. Attempt to understand what went wrong, *own your part in it*, and aim to pull yourself out of what happened better informed—and ready to find a stronger professional match with your skills.

Your network can help with job searches, of course, but beware: When you're looking for a new job, the connections you approach—whether they are personal or professional—are usually not interested in rehashing with you what happened at your old one. Keep the details about what happened to no more than a couple of sentences: "It wasn't a good match" or "I felt the pull of other opportunities." Don't talk trash about places and people, because the world can be awfully small.

Starting fresh gives you a chance to think long and hard about what you'd like to do next. Consider what you loved about previous jobs—as well as what aspects didn't excite you as much. Knowing what you want out of a job—and what you have to offer—is a great first step toward focusing your efforts.

Follow these steps for a successful job search:

1. Write a professional development plan to focus your efforts (see Lesson 41). This plan will help you recognize your strengths, identify target organizations, and begin your networking efforts. Then list 20 places where you'd like to work. Keep your list dynamic—if you cross off a company that's no longer a contender, replace it with another.

2. Update your résumé (see Lesson 42), seeking help from a mentor, a human resources professional, or other experts. But beware of conflicting advice from different sources, and don't spend too much time on your résumé's content because, although important, a résumé is only a tool. It's who you are, what you offer, and your professional experiences—not endless wordsmithing—that will land you the job. Get your one-pager set, and then begin pounding the pavement.

3. Begin networking within and around your list of top 20 organizations (see Lesson 43). After you identify the positions that fit your levels of education and experience, attempt to understand each organization's structure. Who does the hiring? Which of your contacts has some link to that person? Even tangential relationships can open the door a crack. Submitting a formal application will make you just another applicant in a teeming sea of qualified and unqualified hopefuls. Your network can help you stand out, upping your chances that you'll get in the door for an interview.

   A word of caution: Don't think you can rely solely on e-mail and the Internet to land a job. You'll need to reach out and meet with people every day. Unnerving as personal contacts can be, even a follow-up cold call (practiced beforehand, of course) is better than a tiresome e-mail with attachments that may never be opened. Show you care by putting yourself out there—you'll be among the few who do.

4. Practice and prepare for initial interviews that may be conducted by phone. Coach yourself, and cultivate your telephone demeanor as well as a series of short, succinct bullet points about your personal brand so that you'll be prepared, even if you're given only a few moments.

5. Take time to fully prepare for your face-to-face interview, the most important part of the job search (see Lesson 45). Be ready to show how you can solve the company's problems, remembering to project energy as you explain why the job is a good fit for you and how you'll add remarkable value to the company. Even if you don't get the offer straightaway, you'll leave a lasting impression if you do well and may be remembered and considered for other positions that arise. Never burn any bridges—be respectful and act like a grownup when you *don't* win.

6. Balance aggressiveness in your job search with professionalism and courtesy. If your call or e-mail has not been returned, follow up—but use good judgment to make sure you are coming across as persistent and interested, not as irritating, angry, or pushy.

7. Know how to receive a job offer and negotiate your salary. Your goal is to obtain viable job offers. Never turn down an offer until it is extended. Know what you are worth, and conduct a good-faith negotiation to achieve a fair salary.

Among the most critical components of a job search is keeping your spirits buoyed despite some inevitable setbacks. Keep your emotions steady, and remain focused. Focus, prepare, and move!

EXERCISE 1

Set a goal to write your professional development plan, finish your résumé, and begin networking within the next 30 days. If you're conducting a job search while unemployed, set and achieve specific daily goals. Commit to making a specific number of calls and network connections each day as well as to sending out a certain number of résumés. Read up on companies you're targeting to get a full sense of what they're like, what their priorities are, and what directions they're moving in.

EXERCISE 2

Develop and work with your network. Actively strive to meet with people each day. Most executive jobs come from networking.

RESOURCES

Aldrich, J. 2013. *Climbing the Healthcare Management Ladder: Career Advice from the Top on What It Takes to Succeed.* Baltimore: Health Professions Press.

American College of Healthcare Executives. 2014. "Careers." Accessed November 11. www.healthmanagementcareers.org /careers.cfm.

About the Authors

Kenneth R. White, PhD, APRN-BC, FACHE, FAAN, is the University of Virginia (UVA) Medical Center endowed professor of nursing and associate dean for strategic partnerships and innovation in the School of Nursing at UVA. He also holds joint appointments in the UVA Darden School of Business and McIntire School of Commerce. Ken has more than 40 years' experience in healthcare organizations in clinical, administrative, governance, and consulting capacities. He spent 13 years with Mercy Health Services as senior executive in marketing, operations, and international healthcare consulting. From 1995 to 2001, Ken was associate director of the Master of Health Administration and Master of Science in Health Administration programs at Virginia Commonwealth University (VCU), and from 2001 to 2008, he was director of VCU's Master of Health Administration program. He served from 2006 to 2009 as VCU's first Charles P. Cardwell, Jr., Professor and from 2012 to 2013 as VCU's inaugural Sentara Healthcare Professor of Health Administration.

Ken is a board-certified acute care nurse practitioner with a specialty in palliative care. He is a Fellow of the American Academy of Nursing as well as a Fellow, former Regent, and former member of the Board of Governors of the American College of Healthcare Executives (ACHE). He holds visiting professor appointments at the LUISS Guido Carli University in Rome, Italy, and the Swiss School of Public Health in Lugano, Switzerland.

Ken received a PhD in health services organization and research from VCU. He earned an MPH in health administration at the

University of Oklahoma, an MS in nursing at VCU, and a post-master's certificate in the acute care nurse practitioner program at UVA. He has extensive experience in hospital administration and consulting, particularly in the areas of leadership development, marketing, facility planning, and operations management.

He is coauthor (with John R. Griffith) of *The Well-Managed Healthcare Organization,* fifth, sixth, seventh, and eighth editions; *Thinking Forward: Six Strategies for Successful Organizations;* and *Reaching Excellence in Healthcare Management* (all published by Health Administration Press). Ken is a contributing author to the books *Human Resources in Healthcare: Managing for Success* (Health Administration Press), *Advances in Health Care Organization Theory* (Jossey-Bass), *Perianesthesia Nursing: A Critical Care Approach* (Saunders), *Introduction to Health Services* (Delmar), *Evidence-Based Management in Healthcare* (Health Administration Press), and *Managerial Ethics in Healthcare: A New Perspective* (Health Administration Press).

In 2013, Ken was named one of 120 Visionary Leaders as part of VCU School of Nursing's 120th anniversary celebration. Ken received the ACHE Edgar C. Hayhow Award for Article of the Year in 2006 and the James A. Hamilton Award for Book of the Year in 2012. He has served on several hospital, health system, and community nonprofit boards.

Ken lives in Richmond, Virginia, and Afton, Virginia, with his spouse, Dr. Carl Outen.

J. Stephen Lindsey, MHA, FACHE, has been a principal with Ivy Ventures, LLC, since 2003 and focuses on growth opportunities and business development. Before joining Ivy Ventures, he served as the CEO of HCA Henrico Doctors' Hospital in Richmond, Virginia, for many years and held the position of chairman of Manorhouse Retirement Centers. He is an adjunct professor in the Department of Health Administration at Virginia Commonwealth University (VCU), where he taught executive skills and coordinated the residency program for a number of years. Prior to entering the healthcare field, he was an infantry officer in the US Army.

Steve earned a bachelor of science degree in finance at Louisiana State University. He also holds a master's in health administration from Georgia State University. Steve is a Fellow of the American College of Healthcare Executives (ACHE) and, in 2001, received the ACHE Regent's Award for Virginia executive of the year. He is also an honorary alumnus of the VCU Department of Health Administration.

Steve has been a founder of several start-up healthcare companies. He speaks and writes regularly about early career development and other areas of interest to C-suite executives. Steve is also a cofounder of the LinkedIn group Healthcare C-Suite, whose membership consists of nearly 3,000 carefully screened senior healthcare leaders and healthcare management students.

Steve lives in Richmond, Virginia, with his wife Miriam. He has two children and three grandchildren. He has served on the board of directors of the Bon Secours Foundation and is president of the board of directors of CrossOver Healthcare Ministry.